The Dementia Tool Box ™

A Common Sense Approach
to
Dementia Prevention
and
Brain Wellness

Gary G. Adams

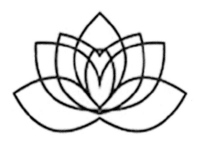

The Dementia Tool Box - The Preview

To know dementia you must experience its devastating effects first hand. Either caring for a loved one who has this impairment, working in a retirement residence, caring facility, or feeling the effects yourself of early memory loss and dementia.

To be told there is no cure is devastating, freighting and heart breaking to be sure.

Let me provide a preview of what you will find in these pages. First the introduction where I explain the signs and symptoms, what is dementia, the crisis, memory workshop, occupations, lifestyles, a lazy brain, cognitive education, recovery and wellness determination.

We then explore the solution, **The Dementia Tool Box** and how each tool is important in preventing or delaying dementia. How the 12 tools working in totality will have a positive impact on this brain impairment.

In the remaining pages we provide a dementia world overview, dementia stories, brain exercises, living longer, stimulating projects and reinforcements.

I encourage everyone to open their Tool Box and begin their dementia defensive program now. I urge you to live a dementia free, brain healthy life. Dementia defense should start in mid-life age 40 to 45. Yes, it is true, life expectancy will soon be 95 and many will live with dementia for 30 years.

AdLinks
Publishing & Marketing
All rights reserved

ISBN: #978-0-9688465-2-0

The information in this publication is not intended to serve
as a replacement for professional medical advice or assistance.
Any use of the information in this publication is at the readers
discretion. The author and the printer specifically disclaim any
and all liability arising directly or indirectly from the use or
application of any information contained herein. References
are made to a number of internet sites; at the time of this
writing, these sites to the best of the author's and/or the printer's knowledge did not contain material that might be offen-
sive to general standard of decency.

THE DEMENTIA TOOLBOX TM

Special discounts are available for bulk purchases
of this book.
For information please contact Special Sales
adamsoriginals@shaw.ca

To purchase individual books please visit
www.mindandmemory.ca

Maintaining a positive attitude,
and being inquisitive
can work wonders, adding
healthful years to your life,
a spring in your step
and a sparkle to your eyes.

Gary Adams

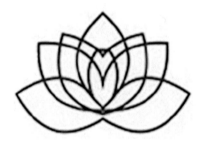

CONTENTS (1)

Welcome

Dementia Tool Box

The 12 Tools

Happiness is nothing more than
good health and real friendships.

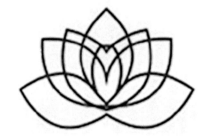

CONTENTS (2)

Introduction (1)

This book is about Dementia Prevention, it is not about Alzheimer's disease. I believe Alzheimer's disease is a hereditary brain disorder. Current studies underway in the United States are researching communities in Brazil where Alzheimer's disease has been widespread and has proven to be passed down from   generation to generation based on years of church records.

In the past 10 years I have presented Mind and Memory Workshops, worked with seniors and consulted with retirement wellness directors, personal aides and on-site medical staff. I have determined that dementia for most people can be prevented by avoiding isolation, being socially active, and constantly exercising the brain. There are 12 defense tools in each person's 'Dementia Tool Box'. They are reviewed in considerable detail in this book.

The Dementia Tools can be applied by anyone at any age (preferably starting at age 40 or even younger) and should be included in an individual's daily routine.

The need for social interaction doesn't change as we age. In fact, it may become even more important (to thriving at an advanced age) than diet or exercise. Loneliness can lead to depression and increased negative emotions. Both are risk factors for dementia. Social isolation causes heightened sensitivity to social threats as well as to self-protective and self-defeating thoughts.

Introduction (2)

Determination

Dementia is a Brain Disorder that can be avoided provided the individual makes a commitment to prevent or reverse this tragic impairment. There is no medical cure and the individual does control his or her own destiny.

Most of Us May Remember smoking and desperately wanting to quit, or being a little or a lot overweight and wanting to lose those extra pounds, but how to get started? We had to set a goal, we had to have absolute determination.

Dementia Requires a Similar Determination. Everyone wants to avoid dementia early or later in life. It is not a disease, but a brain disorder which usually begins with intermittent memory loss. We may live a normal healthy life, then suddenly we begin to forget a phone number, lose are car keys or forget the name of the next door neighbor. This may be a sign of our early stage dementia.

Everyone is potentially on the Pathway That May Lead to Dementia. It is similar to smoking which can lead to lung cancer, excessive weight can lead to heart and stroke disease and hockey and football play can lead to serious brain damage. These are all dreaded health and wellness problems which could have been avoided with a committed life plan.

1. **We Must Set a Goal**. Living an entire life without ever having dementia.

Introduction (3)
Determination

2. **We Must be Specific**, resolutions and goals are useless if there is no commitment. We must follow a specific routine.

3. **We Must Recognize the Potential 'Fall Back'**. "Oh, I have stopped smoking but a few cigars on my birthday should not matter." When on a weight control program, "Oh, A little chocolate cake won't hurt". We must identify the fall backs, and keep an eye on the objective to live a healthy social, brain-wellness life.

4. **We Must Follow the Lifelong Goal** every day, again be specific, make a commitment day by day, week by week, month by month, year by year. Review progress consistently and continue to be open to challenges. Possibly expand education or learn new brain stretching games. Make dementia prevention a lifelong goal.

5. **We Must Celebrate Success**, make new friends, join a new club, take up an interesting hobby and live a happier more fulfilled life.

6. **Live a Lifetime of Wellness**. The years pass more quickly than we could have ever imagined. We wake up one day and we are suddenly older. With a determined goal, an absolute commitment, we can enjoy a better life. We can prevent the pain, confusion and loss of control caused by dementia.

What is Dementia ?

Dementia is a brain disorder, a condition of persistent impairment in brain. It is a group of symptoms associated with a decline in activities, like memory, thinking or speaking. Severe enough to interfere with daily life. Symptoms can also include forgetfulness, confusion and the inability to solve routine problems.

Dementia is often wrongly referred to as 'senility' which reflects the formerly widespread but incorrect belief that serious mental decline is a normal part of aging.

If an individual does not build defenses, dementia will continually advance, which means the conditions will gradually get worse as more brain cells deteriorate and are unable to perform.

Many people have memory loss issues. This does not mean they have dementia. There are different causes of memory loss. If you or a loved one is having bouts of memory loss I recommend you visit a doctor to explore the reason.

normal brain   dementia brain

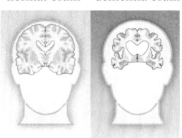

Learn to enjoy every minute
of your life, be happy now.
Smile in the mirror every morning.
Don't complicate things,
avoid stress,
just enjoy life!

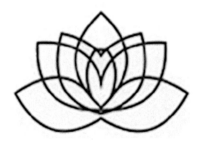

A Growing Crisis

Dementia is a growing crisis. At age 75, sixteen percent of the North American population will have some form of dementia. Without continuous brain care at age 85 one third of the population will have dementia.

If there are no changes in the way we address this brain disorder the number of people who will need dementia care during the next 20 to 50 years will exceed the financial ability of most countries to provide care. In the near future there will be a shortage of dementia care facilities (government sponsored apartments). Families will be faced with enormous problems, caring for a dementia affected loved one at home.

In the year of this publication (2019), each day 1,000 Canadians and 10,000 Americans turn 65 years of age. The older population (age 65 plus) will soon outnumber the number of children (age 14 and under).

As a high percentage of the aged will be living with dementia, the costs which will to be passed down to the younger generation will be enormous.

Retirement residences and sponsored
care facilities are now providing
continuing daily programs
to repair and stimulate
the brains of their residents.

Constant brain activity and
brain challenges are the keys
to controlling and potentially
reversing dementia.

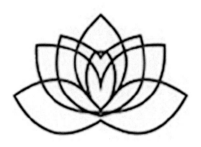

Potential Causes of Memory Loss

Antidepressants, antihistamines

Medications for anxiety medications, tranquilizers

Head injury

Stroke

Excessive use of sleeping pills

Pain medications

Excessive alcohol

Tobacco

Drug use

Depression and Anxiety

Stress, lack of sleep

Overactive thyroid gland

Dementia Signs and Symptoms

- Memory loss
- Impaired judgment
- Difficulties with abstract thinking
- Faulty reasoning
- Inappropriate behavior
- Loss of communication skills
- Disorientation
- Gait motor and balance problems
- Neglect of personal care and safety
- Repeatedly asking the same question
- Hallucinations
- Disoriented in familiar places
- Unable to follow directions
- Confused about the time of day
- Unable to recognize familiar people
- Difficulty with routine skills

Is Dementia Simply a Lazy Brain ?

What causes a person to have Dementia Disorder?

It is said, it is not a disease.

It is not hereditary.

It is not common among highly educated people.

It is not common among people who had brain challenging employment, professions or active lifestyles.

It is very common among people who live with little or no social involvement.

It is very common among people who retire and have few brain stimulating interests.

It is very common among people who live in isolation.

Currently there are 55 million people worldwide affected with dementia and 10 million being added each year. It is therefore not restricted by world region.

The question ... Is Dementia simply
A Lazy Brain ?

Research suggests that the human brain must have continuing exercise and stimulation to remain healthy.

If not, it will slowly shrink, lose memory and lose its ability to function properly.

Prevention

The common question being asked, "if I have a mental, social and physically active life will I avoid dementia?" My observations and experiences suggest that those people who are more socially active, have a much lower chance of developing dementia   disorders. This does not provide absolute proof, but there is growing belief that healthy bodies and active brains combined with higher levels of social activity can delay or totally eliminate the onset of dementia.

I have hosted hundreds of audience presentations that strongly confirm my belief that proper education in early life never-ending study and learning as an adult are a major factor in maintaining brain resilience and brain wellness.

My workshops suggest that early retirement with no real on-going interests or activities can then lead to the slippery slope of brain disorder. There is little question that the brain needs a regular dose of mind stimulating activity. We now know people who retire and then make television their main activity will likely find the brain begins to suffer.

Similarly those of ill health, such as bed ridden patients who watch endless amounts of television instead of reading or practicing brain puzzles and other brain stimulating challenges, will likely experience brain complications.

Dementia Memory Workshops

My dementia prevention / memory workshops, normally include 30 to 50 people who are determined to exercise their brains. Our objective is to delay or prevent dementia by providing weekly brain exercises which stimulate, energize and challenge the brain. Over these past 10 years we have coached hundreds of senior participants mostly in their 70s, 80s, 90s and some over 100 years of age. Those who participate are   working to preserving a healthy active brain.

In addition our workshops have included partners, wives, husbands, adult children, friends and aides. The workshops include Mind and Memory challenging questions the audience responds using hand held devices. The on-screen multiple choice questions and answers, and scores are immediately provided.

I am continually consulting with retirement resident wellness directors and aides who encourage dementia victims to participate in these programs. We have been able to compare the lives of those who participate in our memory programs with those who for the most part have given up and live in isolation. Unfortunately there are thousands who, when they start to lose their memory and recognize dementia is overtaking their mind, simply give up. **Our challenge is to encourage everyone to fight this disorder and use all the tools in their 'Dementia Tool Box'.**

Early Stages (1)
Questionnaire

The following questionnaire may serve as a tool to determine if your loved one is showing signs of dementia.

1. Does your loved one have memory loss?

2. If yes, is his or her memory loss worse than a few years ago?

3. Does your loved one repeat questions, statements or stories the same day?

4. Does your loved one forget about appointments or events?

✓ 5. Does your loved one misplace items and can't find them?

6. Does your loved one suspect others of stealing or hiding items when she/he can't find them?

✓ 7. Does your loved one frequently have trouble knowing the day, month, year or time, or have to repeatedly check the date?

8. Does your loved one have trouble handling money?

9. Does your loved one have trouble paying bills or counting change?

10. Does your loved one have trouble remembering to take medicines?

✓ 11. Does your loved one have trouble with kitchen appliances or setting an alarm clock?

✓ 12. Does your loved one have trouble with common tasks such as operating counter top appliances or vacuum cleaners?

Early Stages Questionnaire (2)

13. Does your loved one frequently become disoriented in unfamiliar places ?

14. When driving, does your loved one lose his/her way ?

15. Does your loved one have trouble concentrating ?

Interpreting Scores

0 to 4 – No cause for alarm

5 to 10 – Memory loss may be an early warning sign

11 to 14 – Early dementia is likely occurring

15 dementia disorder has likely developed

Dementia Recovery

Recovery is possible, but the difficulty lies in motivating the individual to make the commitment. Defining a set of goals, and instilling a determination to fight this disorder. Recovery must include a daily commitment.

Recovery is not an event that happens in a single moment. It is a journey that takes place over a period of time. Sometimes the memory quickly sharpens or it may take weeks or months. However, it all starts with a firm and committed decision to live with a healthy mind and memory. It needs the support of family, friends and possibly an employer. For most people in stage one or two, dementia can be reversed and the individual can return to a meaningful life. In stage 4 recovery is unlikely.

Normal Brain   Dementia Brain

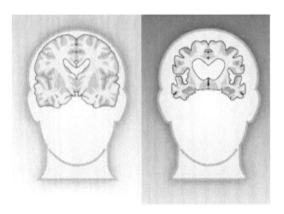

Statistics

- Statistics clearly show that a higher percentage of women are diagnosed with dementia than men.
- There are at least 5.5 million North Americans living with dementia. Of these approximately 3.6 million (65%) are women.
- The total number of North Americans with dementia disorders will rise to 7.5 million by the year 2030 and 10 to 13 million will be living with dementia by the year 2050.
- It is a fact women in their 60s are twice as likely to develop dementia than will develop either breast cancer or heart disease.
- Historically when family illness occurs, the woman is the caregiver. Now she will likely be the patient and the family is living with a frightening experience which will involve a commitment of serious amounts of time and money.
- Depression is a major factor in developing dementia and women are far more susceptible to depression than men.
- It is commonly assumed that women live longer and therefore dementia is more prevalent in women
- Non-working mothers and possibly fathers who may have less opportunity or time to advance their knowledge and expand their social lives are more commonly subject to dementia.

Dementia Medical Treatments

While a medical cure is unknown, victims of dementia are commonly living for 10 to 20 more years once diagnosed and will need continuous home or institutional care.

Unfortunately the grasp of the genetics of dementia, the ability to detect and diagnose these disorders earlier and the development of new compounds to act as treatments are still in their infancy. Scientists are working in most major countries but unless there is a major breakthrough, no medical cure is anticipated in the near future. The brain is very complex.

It is commonly accepted that dementia is not inherited. The answer for most of the population is that our family history is not responsible for this condition.

High blood pressure, obesity, high cholesterol and diabetes are all risk factors for dementia. People with these conditions in mid-life are possibly twice as likely on average to develop dementia later in life.

Note: Wealthy individuals including Ted Turner and Bill Gates whose families have been affected by dementia or Alzheimer's disease have donated millions of dollars for research. This research continues in most major world countries.

24

Adopting a positive attitude can
make dreams come true.

Marion Morrison

Lifestyles — Occupations

Occupations found to help preserve healthy brain function are those which:

- Require complex thinking

- Require communication with people

- Require team work

- That are connected with music

- That require creativity

- That require constant study and upgrading

- That require public presentations

- That involve community fundraising

- That require leadership

Specific Occupations That Commonly Avoid Dementia

Scientists

Managers

Teachers

Educators

Lawyers

Bankers

Doctors

Nurses

Engineers

Accountants

Dentists

Tech code writers

Researchers

Pharmacists

Waitresses

Waiters

Sales people

Reporters

Commentators

Authors

Publishers

Entertainers

Comedians

Actors

Musicians

Artists

Lifestyles of Individuals Most Susceptible to Dementia:

Mothers and fathers without social connections

Criminals living in institutions

People in permanent care or hospitals

Isolated residents living in retirement centers

Women or men working in isolation

Jobs with low decision requirements

Manual work

Store stackers

Long haul truck drivers

Garbage collectors

Laborers

Janitors / cleaning

Night watchmen

High physical demands (with low occupational demands)

Repetitious assembly line workers

Door to door flyer and newspaper distributors

What is Cognitive Reserve ?

To further understand dementia we can look at cognitive reserve. Cognitive reserve is the Bank of Knowledge you use every day at work and in life.

Cognitive skills are the core skills the brain uses to think, read, learn, remember, reason and pay attention. The word 'cognitive' means 'thinking and awareness'. The inner workings of the mind and how they affect the human experience.

Cognitive skills play an important part in processing new information. That means if even one of these skills is weak, no matter what information is coming your way, grasping, retaining, or using that information is impacted. In fact, most learning struggles are caused by one or more weak cognitive skills.

Required cognitive skills:

Long term memory

Short term memory

Remembering why you are doing a current project

Understanding

Knowing the difference

Knowing how to express thoughts

Understanding communication

Understanding reasons why

Time perception

Cognitive Skills

Remember information while doing two things at once.

Remember to recall information stored in the past.

Expressive communication

Learn how to perform a task

Pay attention to a specific subject

Analyze, blend and recognize sounds

Perform tasks quickly and accurately

Learn and comprehend information

Remain calm

Control stress

Be creative for a short term plan

Think before taking action

Think about unexpected changes

Understand

Solve problems

Think outside the box

Have social skills

Have visual images

Cognitive Reserve, Education

Being educated, having higher levels of social interaction or working in cognitively demanding occupations increases resilience to cognitive decline and the risk of dementia.

Higher education is associated with better health and longer life expectancy. Advanced education enhances a person's cognitive skills including literacy, numeracy, and problem-solving skills, enabling them to perform more complex tasks.

Those without proper education have the greater risk of developing impairments in the area of cognitive function, such as memory, reasoning and verbal ability as they age. They have a greater risk of dementia, which is recognized as cognitive decline that interferes with daily life

It is a well known fact that the extent of a person's cognitive decline doesn't occur in line with the amount of biological damage in their brain as it ages. Decline in cognitive function is often the lack of brain use or brain exercise. This may be simply a lazy or seldom challenged brain.

Random Brain Facts (1)

- The brain needs physical exercise.

- The brain needs mental stimulation to remain healthy.

- In a healthy brain memory storage is unlimited.

- The brain is more active while asleep than when watching television.

- The size of the brain has no affect on intelligence.

- Being inquisitive energizes the brain.

- Social isolation can create major health problems.

- The brain is 73% water and takes only 2% dehydration to affect attention, memory and other cognitive skills.

- Ninety minutes of sweating will temporarily shrink the brain.

- Morning dreams can last 30 to 45 minutes.

- Brains are negatively impacted by cell phones and other electronic devices.

- The average brain of an adult weighs about 3.3 pounds.

- The brain contains about 86 billion nerve cells (neurons).

- The brain comprises, on average, about 2% of total body weight, but uses 20% of its total energy and oxygen intake.

Random Brain Facts (2)

- Music triggers activity in the same brain structure that releases the 'pleasure chemical' dopamine during sex and eating.

- Cognitive is the mental act or process by which knowledge is acquired.

- A scan of a famous singer and artist's brain found that composing music, writing poetry and creating art activates different parts of the brain.

- Even a short, one-time burst of exercise can boost brain function such as decision-making focus.

- A study using MRI scans show brains of people who exercise moderately look 10 years younger than those who do not.

- A person with an active healthy brain can have about 70,000 thoughts each day.

The Brain

The average brain weighs 3.3 pounds and has

100,000 miles of blood vessels.

It is often said the brain contains more connections

than stars in the sky.

Your brain could be suffering this very minute and

you may not have a clue.

Normal   Severe Dementia

I Am Dementia

I will take possession of your Mind and Memory, often in your younger years. I will begin my work, slowly creeping, disconnecting more and more of your brain cells, upsetting your cognitive skills.

Yes, I am a nasty brain-altering disorder. I will eliminate your ability to think clearly, read, learn, remember, listen to reason and pay attention. I normally enter your brain when you are in your younger years. You will probably not notice that I have arrived. Depending on your lifestyle I will initially begin my work with no noticeable effect on your daily routine.

When you reach age 40 to 75 and have had an inactive brain life or have decided to retire your brain, I will activate my four stage program. In the beginning I will concentrate on your memory, you will forget names, lose your football game tickets, and forget your love partner's birthday.

During the next several years I will gradually, totally dismantle your brain, you will not be able to communicate with others, understand where you are, recognize friends and family, travel or drive your car. I intend to spend 20 years or more disrupting your brain, and you won't remember how it happened.

Author: Gary G. Adams

There is no known medical cure for
Dementia. But I believe the lifestyle choices
presented in the Dementia Tool Box
in the following pages can
reverse or delay impairment to the brain.

Gary G. Adams

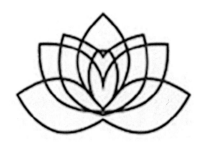

Dementia Tool Box

1. Be Socially Active
2. Be Brain Healthy
3. Concentrate on Memory
4. Exercise Daily
5. Eat Healthfully
6. Avoid Isolation
7. Be a Constant Learner
8. Manage Stress
9. Live a Happy Life
10. Encourage Laughter
11. Be Musically Inspired
12. Refresh and Energize

THE DEMENTIA TOOLBOX TM

Dementia Tool Box (1)

The Dementia Tool Box which contains twelve tools which can be activated to avoid, delay or reverse dementia brain disorder.

I firmly believe that one good choice will not have any serious impact on dementia, but the totality of 12 self imposed **Dementia Tools in the Tool Box** can make a tremendous difference.

Dementia is a brain disorder which needs constant attention from an early age. We must care for and exercise our brain as we live our daily lives.

The tools are listed in order of importance. The first three tools, (a socially active life, having a healthy active brain, and constantly concentrating on memory techniques) are all critical in order to avoid dementia.

All of the tools in our **Dementia Tool Box** are significant, which include daily exercise, eating healthfully, expanding   education, avoid stress, live a happy engaged life, encourage laughter, listen to music to nourish our brain and live a refreshed, energized life and most importantly avoid isolation.

Dementia Tool Box (2)

Let us begin to explore these twelve tools and examine the importance of each. Our readers likely range from age 30 to possibly 100 plus. The majority will recognize but they or their loved ones are heading into an age bracket where dementia is prevalent. They will also discover they have friends who may already be showing early signs of dementia disorder. Others will also recognize these early warnings may have been present in their brains.

For those as young as 30, the 'Tool Box' is most important. Start now to expand a social life. Use brain exercises and practice brain techniques daily. Brain exercise is equally important as physical exercise.

If you have not had a socially active life, not had regular brain challenges and have not practiced memory programs, you should start now.

START RIGHT NOW
Avoid Dementia,
Live a Happy, Healthier Life.

All the adversity I've had in my life,
all my troubles and obstacles,
have strengthened me.
You may not realize it when
it happens but it may be the best
thing in the world for you.

Walt Disney

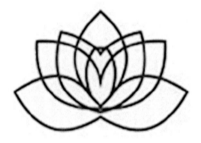

Tool #1
Be Socially
Active

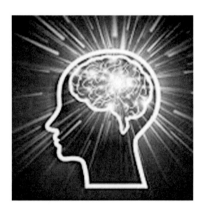

Be Socially Active (1)

Socializing is extremely important to build a defense against dementia. It is absolutely critical for people of all ages to make the extra effort to maintain relationships with friends, neighbors, and relatives, as well as to encourage new friendships as we age. It is the time to recognize the growing importance of expanding our social lives.

Feelings of loneliness and social isolation can be common amongst older adults, especially those who may have lost their partners or a close friend. It may seem difficult due to our age, health or financial conditions to find ways to make new friends and stay active in the community. There are many community organizations that offer events and programs to improve older adults physical and mental health.

Take the first step to expand your social life. Don't wait for others to initiate conversation. Remember to be a serious listener, people love to talk about themselves.

Jump start, make decisions. Be the person who says "Let's do this today". Suggest a dinner out, attend free events, make it happen. Use creativity to encourage outings that you and your friends will enjoy. Spend time researching stimulating, interesting events.

Be Socially Active (2)

Stress and feelings of isolation caused by issues with family or finances often intensify depression, anxiety and dementia. Social interaction and continued participation combats depression and improves confidence and well being.

People who maintain valued relationships tend to live longer and live healthier lives, but it takes a little effort, a phone call, meeting some friends for breakfast. Make it an event and include several friends. Select a topic for discussion for each week.

Socializing with people is an easy but intricate challenge. Organize a coffee club to be held at a different home each week. Have each person bring a friend. Keep it simple and offer healthy snacks.

Connect on social media, such as e-mail, Face Book and Twitter which are popular with all ages. It is easy to connect with family and friends and to reconnect with people from your past. Search for high school or university friends. Establish a game night, play cards or other popular games. Encourage everyone to bring a friend. Play Wizard, the #1 group (4 to 6 players) dementia   prevention card game which provides excellent brain strategy and stimulation.

Be Socially Active (3)

It's not unexpected for people to become socially isolated as they age, as family dynamics change. Make an effort to explore new opportunities. Become involved in activities that demand interaction.

Social activities keep us sharp and mentally engaged which is extremely important. Connecting with others helps keep you in a positive mood which in turn wards off depression and negative thoughts. It has been determined that people who participate with others, maintain real lifelong friendships, will live a happier life as they age.

The following suggestions provide ways to expand your social life and encourage new friendships:

- Meet the merchants in your area
- Give someone a gift for no obvious reason
- Have a barbeque and invite the neighbors
- Invite someone you just met to a sporting event
- Join a social or hobby club
- Join a fitness group or yoga class
- Join toastmasters, become a public speaker
- Join Creative Retirement
- Organize a Wizard card group, play regularly

Be Socially Active (4)

- Learn new dance routines
- Join a limerick or poetry authors club
- Organize a weekly breakfast group
- Walk and talk with a friend
- Participate in community fund raising events
- Attend art classes
- Become an author and write 'My Life Story'
- Participate in a 'Crochet and Chat' group
- Join a camera club
- Play sports that involve team play
- Like to sing. Join a choir
- Learn to play a musical instrument
- Learn to play brain stretching card games
- Adopt a pet and connect with a training class
- Play pickle ball or golf
- Join an actor's group, learn how to be a new you
- Attend lectures, learn about a new subject
- Offer to be on a community board of directors
- Learn to play chess or bridge
- Participate in Mind & Memory events

**A Thriving Social Life Will Do Wonders for
Your Mind and Your Body**

Be Socially Active (5)

- Join a Seniors' Club
- Join a Veterans' Club
- Join a Creative Cooking Club
- Learn an alternative language
- Attend history classes
- Attend an educational lecture
- Learn the art of Origami
- Attend a pottery class
- Attend a wood carving class
- Learn new computer programs
- Join an e-mail joke club
- Take a photography course
- Join a walking tour group
- Complete crossword puzzles
- Attend challenging fun trivia programs
- Attend an investment workshop
- Take music lessons
- Join a wine tasting club
- Attend an educational movie
- Attend armchair travel presentations

Tool #2
Healthy Brain

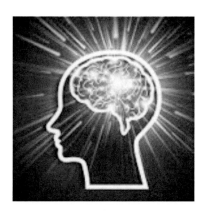

Healthy Active Brain (1)

When people of all ages keep their minds active, their thinking and memory skills are less likely to decline. Mind games, puzzles, trivia memory challenges and other types of brain training will help slow memory loss, forgetfulness and other disorders.

Brain exercises may vary from person to person. The main idea is to keep your brain active and challenged. Start with something as simple as eating with the hand you don't normally use or read a paragraph or two backwards. You might also:

- Build social networks live or on-line
- Avoid depression, care for your emotions
- Make it your goal to learn something new every day
- Learn to play competitive bridge, chess or wizard
- Join a group that plays on a regular weekly schedule
- Learn to take professional or at least better photographs
- Build the biggest and toughest table puzzles
- Become an expert on movies, actors, when they were introduced, and who won Oscars
- Pick a subject and write a presentation which you are supposedly going to present to an audience of 50 people
- Write a book, everyone has at least one book in them
- Learn about computer programs and teach others

Healthy Active Brain (2)

It is a fact, exercise improves brain function and repairs damaged brain cells. The part of the brain that responds strongly to physical exercise is the hippocampus. Well controlled experiments in children, adults and the elderly shows that brain structure grows as people become healthier. The hippocampus is at the core of the brain's learning and memory systems. This explains the memory boosting effects of improved cardiovascular fitness.

Evidence confirms that staying physically fit keeps your brain healthy into old age. Workouts need not be extreme. A 30-45 minute brisk walk, three to four times a week can deflect the mental wear and tear and delay the onset of dementia.

Exercise improves balance, coordination and nimbleness making a clear impact on the brain structure and cognitive function. Walking, either on a treadmill or around the neighbor-hood can bolster divergent, creative thinking and memory. Yoga is an amazing tool to stretch and improve flexibility. Yoga can also help focus and quiet the mind.

Don't sit still. Our minds don't operate in isolation. What you do with your body affects on your brain's mental faculties. Sitting still all day, every day, makes you vulnerable. Don't   procrastinate, keep your brain healthy, find something you   enjoy. Just get up and do it.

Healthy Brain Review

The brain changes with age and needs continuing exercises. Here are some suggestions:

- Have regular brain stimulation

- Have ongoing physical exercise

- Improve your diet

- Improve your blood sugar

- Improve your cholesterol

- Stop smoking

- Drink alcohol in moderation

- Control emotions and depression

- Build social networks

- Get proper sleep, including short naps

- On the advise of your doctor, include vitamin D, B12, and CoEnzyme Q10 in your daily diet.

- Follow my accountant's favorite brain exercise. While reading a book or the newspaper, occasionally read a paragraph out loud and backwards.

Expand Your Vocabulary (1)
Exercise the Brain

#1 **Flamenco** is which of the following?
   a. a type of Italian bread
   b. a flame thrower
   c. a dark dream
   d. a type of dance and music

#2 **Requite** is which of the following?
   a. to rewrite a poem
   b. a return for kindness
   c. to advance in age
   d. a poorly drained marsh

#3 **Shive** is which of the following?
   a. a flat cork for wide mouthed bottles
   b. a plant with yellow flowers
   c. an engineering device
   d. a pig that weighs less than 30 pounds

#4 **Grizzled** is which of the following?
   a. a damaged flower
   b. overcooked bacon
   c. a defeated old soldier
   d. grey hair

#5 **Barley** is which of the following?
   a. a course weedy plant
   b. a clip for holding papers
   c. a tobacco
   d. a four stroke engine

Expand Your Vocabulary (2)

#6 **Parry** is which of the following?
a. wonder aloud
b. skillfully avoid a question
c. repeat an answer
d. a form of bridge

#7 **Quaver** is which of the following?
a. whisper
b. speak with a trembling voice
c. describe enthusiastically
d. make a counter argument

#8 **Calumniate** is which of the following?
a. agree without thinking
b. make a false and defamatory statement
c. take a unlikely guess
d. mumble nervously

Vocabulary Answers
1. D
2. B
3. A
4. D
5. C
6. B
7. B
8. B

Subscribe to Readers Digest and include these brain challenges in your brain exercise program.

Tool #3
Memory
Concentration

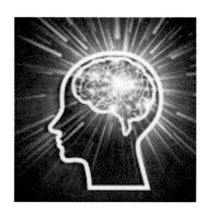

It is better to dance than
to march through life.

Yoko Ono

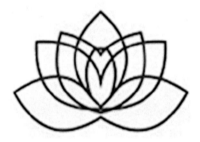

Memory Concentration

As we age it gets harder to concentrate and give our total and undivided attention to the task at hand. Is absolutely critical if we are to have a better memory. Concentrating to the task at hand is absolutely necessary to avoid memory loss or an embarrassing event or happening.

Attention and concentration are critical mental skills. In fact many memory complaints are actually about the failure to concentrate.

Take the example of not remembering where the car is parked after shopping or at the ball game. It is likely that you did not pay much attention to where your car was parked in the first place. The brain is left with few opportunities to register any information that could be recalled later to help find the car. This also applies to keys, the remote and eye glasses.

Focus on the task at hand. If talking with someone, listen and then ask questions. Avoid and eliminate distractions. Tune out everything else. The harder the task the more important it is to concentrate. Turn off the television when answering the telephone.

Resist double-tasking or multi-tasking. This will increase errors and divide attention. By dividing attention unnecessary mistakes could be made. Concentration, motivation and heightened awareness are largely a matter of focus.

Suggested Concentration Exercises:

Make a list of 12 unrelated items, a flower, ketchup, a candle, a chair, a shovel, a clock, a stool, a car, a razor, a mirror, a book and a lamp. Concentrate on the list. Read the list 3 times over then cover the list. Now write the items in the exact order on a separate piece of paper.

Add 6 items to the list (now 18 items) and repeat the foregoing. Return to the list, add two items to your group of 18 (now 20) and from memory write the items on a separate piece of paper. Now, from memory write the list backwards.

Make a list of 12 birds (a little more difficult) a swan, a crow, a sparrow, a hawk, a swallow, a blue jay, an owl, a dove, a warbler, a pigeon, a parrot, and a robin. Concentrate on your list, from memory write the list on a piece of paper.

Add 6 more birds to the list (now 18 birds) and repeat as above. Return to the list, add six more birds (finch, gull, woodpecker, heron, blackbird, flycatcher) to your group of 18 (now 24) and from memory write the birds on a separate piece of paper. Now, from memory write the list of 24 backwards

Suggested Concentration Exercises:

Write 10 given and family names on separate cards. Place the cards in various locations such as on the TV, on the kitchen table, on the counter, etc. Next write a list of locations and then from memory add first and last names. Repeat the foregoing, increasing the list to 16 names, then again with 24 names. Repeat this challenge two days later.

Test Your Brain

Make a list of things to do. A grocery list or recipe or whatever comes to mind. Memorize your list and two hours later write down your list on a pad of paper. Be sure to make it challenging and potentially difficult.

Make a list of 12 challenges multiplications and divisions. All in your head, without the use of a calculator or a pencil resolve these calculations. Try walking or riding a stationery bike at the same time.

Test your concentration, after visiting a new neighborhood, a park or shopping center, draw a map of the area. Expand your thought process. Think of a word with multiple letters and then in your head without references list other words that begin and end with the same letters.

Brain Boosting

Become involved in something new. Attend a workshop or seminar which has audience participation and requires each member to answer questions. It should be based on a subject that is unfamiliar which forces the imagination to be stretched. Not a subject that is recognized. The object is to expand brain skills and learn something new.

Take on a new challenge. A brain-boosting activity such as a publication which features Sudoku or Trivia and demands concentration. It could also be bridge lessons, a computer course, music lessons, a course in embroidery or golf lessons. Make it a regular happening not something that you already know but something that is a real challenge that will demand real focus and effort.

Old habits such as driving the car, tying shoelaces do little to enhance the memory. Find activities, preferably something new and difficult which stretch the brain and memory. Join an art group, learn to blend acrylic paint colors. Did you know there are over 3,000 new English words added to the Oxford Dictionary every year? Put a few new words into your memory bank, make your next e-mail or audience presentation more interesting.

The Memory Bank

Memory is critically important in our day to day lives. Every day we need our memory to help make simple and important decisions. Without a memory bank we would not know how to get dressed, bathe, shave, make the morning coffee, drive the car, or shop for groceries. To live a normal life we must have an active memory bank.

Inability to make decisions based on memory is an example of dementia. A properly functioning memory is absolutely necessary for anyone to live a normal life, to drive to work, know the route, navigate in traffic, take an alternate route if necessary, to fill the car with gas, to have the proper credit card in our wallet or purse. Memory loss makes it impossible to reason, and make everyday decisions.

Those who have early stage dementia, usually find it difficult to absorb new information. They then become more forgetful.

The brain has the ability to adapt, change and learn. With stimulation the brain can create and make new connections. It is important for everyone, regardless of age to have a brain health memory exercise program.

Healthy Brain Review

- Have constant brain stimulation

- Include constant physical exercise

- Improve diet

- Improve blood sugar

- Improve cholesterol

- Ride a stationary bike

- Practice flash cards while peddling

- Play music and sing while peddling

- Manage emotions and depression

- Build social networks

- Proper sleep and short naps

- Practice word puzzles

- Test your vocabulary

- Do spelling puzzles

- Make lists

- Write down new information (make it a habit)

Memory Focus (1)

The Mind and Memory Workshops have proven over and over again that people, regardless of age, who **concentrate** will have stronger memories. The importance of concentration must be emphasized. It is the key. it will unquestionably improve memory.

Building and retaining memory requires focus, from an early age and through ages 45, 50s, 60s, 70s, 80s and 90s. **Focus, Focus, Focus** on what is being discussed or planned. By staying focused the memory will absorb the matter at hand.

Every time you learn something new, take on a new challenge, play a new game or meet new people. Your memory cannot function efficiently if you do not focus.

In the Mind and Memory Workshops concentration is practiced using a focus tool. For an example: The images of 5 clowns appear on the screen. Each clown has a name, the audience must now focus on each image and attempt to determine something unique about the image and to remember the name of the clown. The next screen features one of the images and the names of the 5 clowns. Now the audience must determine which name matches that particular clown. Similar to multiple choice trivia.

Memory Focus (2)

A second example: In the Workshops we illustrate the importance of being focused, the audience will determine what is unique about each person.

The following characters appear on the screen:
Ronald has red hair, Mort is mixing chemicals, Paul is holding a box of pills, Walter has white hair, Bob is wearing braces. Each participant must focus on the images. This Workshop exercise provides focus training and concentration.

Later in the workshop we provide a similar challenge. Different characters. Now the audience must focus and develop their own individual clue and remember each image and the connection.

Brain memory requires **you to use it or lose it.** The more seriously you focus and concentrate on the matter at hand the easier it will become to remember people and information.

Memory Focus (3)

How to meet someone new and remember their name:

Good old fashioned paper and pen will keep you focused on the matter at hand. Focus on the person you have just met, go slow and make sure you give the person proper attention. Remember the person's name and be sure the spelling is correct.

The benefit of writing a name on paper, the old-fashioned way, is real and will make a good impression when a person sees you recording their name.

The smart phone or tablet could be a useful tool to keep a record of names and related information. If handed a business card, thank them and read their name out loud.

Remember this is not about you. Give your full attention to this new acquaintance and concentrate on him or her.

Memory Focus (4)

Seriously caring about the person you meet for the first time is an exceptional memory tool in the **Tool Box**. Be curious, what is this person all about, what is their background, do we have common friends or other connections? What line of work are or were they involved in, do or did we live in the same neighborhood? Do we have common interests? Do we belong to the same clubs or associations?

Pay Attention, **you must pay attention** when you meet someone new if you seriously want to remember their name. Transfer their name from your short term memory to your long term memory. This normally takes about 6 to 8 seconds if you are concentrating. Focus, focus, pay attention to the name and forget about yourself.

Develop a **New Acquaintance Memory Plan**. Keep a small book in the car or hand bag when going to an event or luncheon to record the names of any new acquaintances.

Remember by Association

Memory experts have found that visual association helps to remember names. Develop a visual picture of the person you have met. Does he or she remind you of another person, a bird, a car a product or a topic?

Memory Creativity

Visualize a picture or story in your mind. Names and numbers by themselves can easily be forgotten if there is little or no association involved. As you learn new information, be aware of the surroundings and any details you can later associate with this new information. Recognize the order of events and then you can replay them in your mind to retrieve them later.

Make a Connection

Example: A new credit card security number is #1402. It is the same number of an apartment rented, a license number or other number related device which is easily remembered.   My mother's birthday was the 14th of February (14-02).

Memory Challenge

Example:

This is a list of 8 unrelated words. Set a stop watch for one minute to study the words. Then spend 10 minutes doing something else. Now write down as many words as you can remember.

COW   APPLE   NURSE   CIGAR

FIREMAN   RADIO   FLUTE   YELLOW

Visualizing a story that links unrelated words will automatically boost your recall. Look at the 8 words again and this time visualize a story that links them all together.

Visualize a parade with a fireman with yellow hair eating an apple, listening to a radio while riding a cow, or a nurse smoking a cigar and playing a flute. Use your first associations and link the images in any order. Now write the words again and see how your memory has improved.

LION   ELEPHANT   ACROBAT   BALLOON

CLOWN   DRUM   TRUMPET   FLAG

Visualize a circus with a clown waving a flag, and an acrobat riding an elephant while playing a trumpet, a lion playing a drum and colorful balloons floating in the air. Use your first associations and link the images in any order. Repeat as above.

Memory Exercises

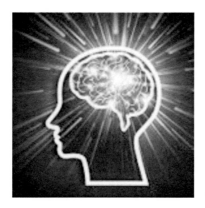

The mind has no limit.
As long as the mind can
envision the fact that you can
do something, you can do it,
as long as you absolutely believe.

Arnold Schwarzenegger

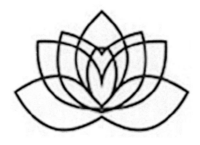

Memory Exercises

The exercises on the following pages provide mind stretching challenging memory puzzles. Take 3 to 5 minutes to memorize each exercise and on a separate pad write down the objects or names by memory which were on the list. Practice each day and improve the memory.

These puzzles are similar to the everyday challenges of   remembering the names of friends, commitments, grocery lists, appointments and a variety of other information. Developing new memory skills will give you confidence to take on new memory challenges all with the objective of avoiding dementia.

Once you have mastered these five exercises, create your own new list, and expand the list to 20 or 30 objects or names. In just one or two weeks you will feel a new confidence about your memory.

Memory Exercise (1)

Take 5 to 10 minutes to memorize these names.
Write the names from memory on a pad of paper.
Repeat this exercise until all the names are memorized.

Suggestion: Divide the names into groups of 3.
Once you have memorized the first 3 names, now add
the next 3 and continue adding 3 names at a time until
you have memorized all 15 names.

Roy
Keith
Morris

Gordon
Peter
Ronald

Donald
George
Richard

Barry
Ernie
Michael

Scott
William
Jackson

Memory Exercise (2)

Take 5 to 10 minutes to memorize these items.
Write the items from memory on a pad of paper.
Repeat this exercise until all the names are memorized.

Suggestion: Divide the items into groups of three.
Once you have memorized the first 3 items, now add
the next 3 and continue adding 3 items at a time until you
have memorized all 15 items.

Button
Tea Pot
Stove

Iron
Spoon
Fry Pan

Table
Toaster
Kettle

Plate
Chair
Fridge

Knife
Plate
Fork

Memory Exercise (3)

Take 5 to 10 minutes to memorize these cities.
Write the cities from memory on a pad of paper.
Repeat this exercise until all the cities are memorized.

Suggestion: Divide the cities into groups of three.
Once you have memorized the first 3 cities, now add
the next 3 and continue adding 3 cities at a time until you
have memorized all 15 cities.

Toronto
New York
London

Paris
Moscow
Vancouver

Las Vegas
Tokyo
Berlin

Melbourne
Sydney
Madrid

Seoul
Washington
Ottawa

Memory Exercise (4)

Take 5 to 10 minutes to memorize these countries.
Write the countries from memory on a pad of paper.
Repeat this exercise until all the countries are memorized.

Suggestion: Divide the countries into groups of three.
Once you have memorized the first 3 countries, now add
the next 3 and continue adding 3 countries at a time until you
have memorized all 15 countries.

Canada
Sweden
France

Mexico
Brazil
Germany

China
India
Finland

Italy
Australia
Columbia

South Korea
Ireland
Netherlands

Memory Exercise (5)

Take 5 to 10 minutes to memorize these names.
Write the names from memory on a pad of paper.
Repeat this exercise until all the names are memorized.

Suggestion: Divide the names into groups of 3.
Once you have memorized the first 3 names, now add
the next 3 and continue adding 3 names at a time until you
have memorized all 15 names.

Tom Anderson
Sheila Brown
Frank Osborne

Mandy Adams
Benda Douglas
George McDonald

Cindy Downing
Louis Chester
Bob Smith

Margaret Webster
Ann Duffer
Sam Penner

Iris Hagland
Norm Jones
Julie Liston

Tool #4
Physical Exercise

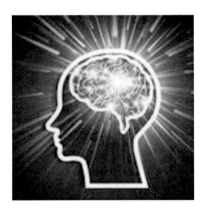

What we become depends on
what we read after all of the
professors have finished with us.
The greatest University of all
is a collection of books

Thomas Carlyle

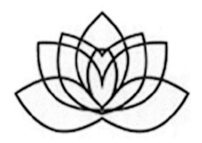

Physical Exercise (1)

If you have been inactive for sometime we recommend you begin your program slowly but with a real commitment ongoing. Remember, some exercise each day is much better than none.

Starting a fitness program may be one of the best things you can do for your health. Make sure you consult your doctor first. Physical activity can reduce your risk of dementia, improve your balance and coordination, help you lose weight and even improve your sleeping habits.

It is an unquestionable fact that a daily exercise routine will strengthen your will to feel better about yourself. Small amounts of physical activity added to your daily, weekly and monthly routine can have an amazing effect on your self esteem.

Choose a simple activity such as 15 to 20 minutes of modest speed walking four times a week. As your confidence builds, increase the speed and distance. It may take a month to make this a habit. Keep a daily journal and record your progress.

If walking alone, make it a time to expand your knowledge. Buy a broadcasting device and rent CD's from your library. If you have a walking partner spend time choosing interesting subjects for discussion. Add some funny stories or one liners!

Build your library of grins and giggles in your memory bank. Everyone loves the person who seems to have a good joke ready for any occasion.

Physical Exercise (2)

What is the right amount of exercise for people with early or middle stage dementia? The Department of Health recommends a regular routine of at least 20 to 45 minutes each day.

Suggestions:

- Ride a stationary bike each day
- Play pickle ball
- Joining the Y, swim and join an exercise class
- Go cycling
- Practice yoga
- Take a regular 30 minute brisk outdoor walk
- Stretch and bend
- Play indoor or lawn bowling
- Play regular or miniature golf
- Play billiards
- Try cross country skiing
- Try snowshoeing
- Use an indoor walking track
- Park the car and walk
- Walk up the stairs instead taking the elevator
- Walk up the stairs instead of the escalator
- Make stair climbing a regular exercise
- Mow the lawn
- Take up gardening

Physical Exercises (1)
For Older Folks

1. Marching is a great balancing exercise for older folks. To start hold on to a steady chair. Stand straight, lift your right knee as high as you can. Lower it, then lift the left leg and lower it. Lift and lower each leg 20 times.

2. Stand at arms length facing the wall. Lean forward slightly and place hands flat against the wall at the height and width of your shoulders. Keep your feet planted as you slowly bring your body towards the wall. Gently push yourself back so that your arms are straight. Repeat 20 times.

3. Stand behind a steady chair with your feet about 3 feet apart. Slowly lift your right leg up to the side. Keep your back straight, your toe facing forward and stare straight ahead. Lower your right leg and repeat with the left leg. Repeat 12 times.

4. Next to a steady chair, stand with your feet together and arms at your sides. Lift your right hand over your head straight up. Then bending your knee lift the right leg so that the upper part of the leg is horizontal. Hold that position for 12 seconds. Repeat the same exercise with the left arm and leg. Repeat 12 times.

5. Seated, rotate your shoulders gently up towards the ceiling, then back and down. Next, do the same thing, but roll them forwards and down. Repeat 9 times with each shoulder.

Physical Exercises (2)
For Older Folks

6. Stand behind a stable heavy chair, hold on to the chair with one hand and lift your right foot up and balance of the left foot for as long as you can. Now reverse your feet. Repeat without holding on to the chair. Repeat 12 times.

7. Walk heel to toe in a straight line. Place the heel of your right foot, touching directly in front of the left foot. Now with the left foot touching and directly in front of the right foot. Then repeat and walk 30 steps. Repeat this exercise 3 times.

8. With feet apart lift the left leg with knee bent, stand for 30 seconds. Repeat and lift your right leg. Repeat exercise 6 times.

9. To stretch the calf muscles, sit on the floor with legs straight out. Place a rope or long towel around the sole of the right foot and hold both ends. Pull the rope or towel towards you while keeping the knee straight and hold for 20 seconds. Repeat 3 times with each leg.

10. Stand with your feet together and arms at your sides. Lift your right leg with knee bent and raise your right arm straight up. Hold for 12   seconds. Repeat this with the left leg and arm. Repeat this exercise 10 times. (If necessary hold on to a chair).

Life expectancy would grow dramatically
if green vegetables smelled as
good as bacon.

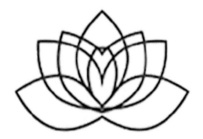

Tool #5
Eat Healthfully

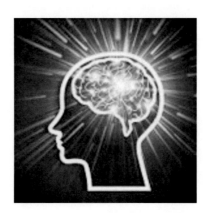

Eat Healthfully (1)

Dementia disorder, like heart and stroke, is linked to saturated fat, cholesterol, and toxins found in meat, dairy products and processed food. People who eat excessive amounts of red meat and dairy products have a greater risk of developing dementia than do vegetarians.

The brain needs fuel. It requires healthy fats, fruits, vegetables, lean proteins, and adequate vitamins and minerals. Consuming too little of these foods and too many complex carbohydrates, processed foods and sugar stimulates the production of toxins in the body. These toxins can lead to inflammation, the build-up of plaque in the brain and can result in impaired cognitive function.

Bread and pasta made with whole grain is higher in B vitamins and minerals, such as copper, selenium and magnesium.

Learn to develop healthy eating habits. Avoid harmful foods. Eat well and exercise to improve your overall health. You will control weight, give yourself a sense of well-being and help boost your energy level. A food-healthy life style will enable you to live longer and potentially avoid the catastrophic effects of dementia. A healthy diet should include fresh vegetables, fruits, lean meats, low fat dairy products plus breads and cereals containing WHOLE GRAINS.

Eat Healthfully (2)

Foods that Help to Boost Memory:

Leafy darker green vegetables

Cruciferous vegetables

Salmon and other cold-water fish

Beans

Spinach

Romaine Lettuce

Kale

Whole Grains

Low Fat Dairy Products

Extra Virgin Olive Oil

Coconut Oil

Celery

Flax Seeds

Cauliflower

Beets

Broccoli

Brussels Sprouts

Eat Healthfully (3)

Fruits that Help to Boost Memory:

Raisins

Blueberries

Blackberries

Strawberries

Raspberries

Plums

Pears

Prunes

Oranges

Apples

Red Grapes

Cherries

Eat Healthfully (4)

Everyone especially those with early dementia should add the following to their daily diet.

Top Antioxidant Foods

Kale

Turmeric

Spinach

Brussels Sprouts

Broccoli Florets

Beets

Corn

Red Peppers

Onions

Eggplant

Chick Peas

Peas

Kidney Beans

Black Beans

Soy Beans

Navy Beans

Pinto Beans

Eat Healthfully (5)
Nuts

Extensive studies confirm that just eating a handful of walnuts each day can stave off the ravages of brain disease. Leading health clinics indicate most nuts are extremely healthy. The following nuts are recommended to help retain brain wellness.

Walnuts

Almonds

Hazelnuts

Pistachios

Cashews

Macadamia

Brazil

Pecans

Peanuts

Processed Foods

A potato comes from the ground, a fruit from a tree or bush, an egg from a hen, but where did that sugar-loaded tart come from? Avoid processed foods which have little if any health benefits.

Processed foods are usually loaded with extra salt and sugar. When grocery shopping select products that are not processed.

Eat Healthfully (6)

It's a fact. Many famous people such as Sir Richard Branson know that tea has many healthy benefits. He drinks 6 to 8 cups a day. It has also been proven that tea drinkers have a lower risk of stroke and heart disease.

Tea has approximately one-half of the caffeine content of coffee. It is less harmful for the heart and doesn't keep you awake at night.

Water, Water, Water, although there are different opinions on how much you should drink most doctors encourage more rather than less. Health experts commonly suggest eight, 8-ounce glasses per day which is about 2 liters.

It is a common belief that if you don't stay hydrated throughout the day, your energy levels and brain function may start to suffer.

The body is 60% to 70% water. You are constantly losing water primarily via urine and sweat. To prevent dehydration you should drink adequate amounts of water each day.

Drinking water helps maintain the balance of body fluids. The function of these body fluids include digestion, absorption, circulation, creation of saliva, transportation of nutrients and maintenance of body temperature.

Through your posterior gland your brain communicates with your kidneys and tells it how much water to excrete as urine or hold for reserves. When you are low on fluids, the brain triggers the body's thirst mechanism. Again indicating the absolute need to have a healthy brain.

Eat Healthfully (7)
Caffeine - The Good and the Bad

The Good

About 40% of studies suggest caffeine has a positive effect on dementia. Caffeine can have a stimulating effect on the central nervous system. The question is how much is too much?

Up to four cups a day is reasonably safe for most healthy adults.

The Bad

Caffeine can increase stress and make you feel ill. If you drink excessive amounts of coffee or drinks containing caffeine, it would not be uncommon to have side effects such as:

> Migraine headaches
>
> Insomnia (lack of sleep)
>
> Nervous stress
>
> Irritability
>
> Frequent urination
>
> Upset stomach
>
> Fast heartbeat
>
> Muscle tremors
>
> Jitters

Caffeine can be dangerous if mixed with certain medications.

Most soft drinks contain caffeine and excessive amounts of sugar.

Eat Healthfully (8)
Reduce Your Sugar Intake

Sugar especially in high doses is a harmful substances. The average North American consumes 140 pounds of sugar each year.

It's a fact. People have trouble believing they are actually consuming that much sugar. Addiction to sugar plays a role in impaired brain function and overall health. Sugar consumed in these quantities is possibly the worst poison you could put into your body.

Symptoms Linked to Excess Sugar Consumption;

- Aggression
- Fatigue
- Increased thirst
- Weight gain
- Increased cholesterol
- Blurred vision
- Headache or stomach ache
- Urination problems
- Dry mouth and skin
- Pain or numbness in your legs

All of the above are harmful as we strive to avoid dementia.

Eat Healthfully (9)
Reduce Your Sugar Intake

Eat plain yogurt with fresh berries

Eat cereals with under 4 grams of sugar per serving

Snack on a banana or apple instead of chocolate

Avoid those pastries, pies and muffins

Choose peanut butter with zero sugar content

Use olive oil on your salad in place of dressings

Replace candy with unsalted nuts

Eat whole unprocessed foods

Snack with a bowl of rolled oats and berries

Avoid all those so called healthy chocolate, fruit and nut bars

Avoid ice cream, have plain yogurt instead

Bananas

Bananas contain dopamine a feel good chemical in your brain

Bananas are rich in fiber

Bananas are rich in antioxidants

Bananas are low in calories, about 105 calories per banana

Bananas are great source of dietary potassium which helps lower blood pressure

Bananas are a weight loss friendly food

Bananas are a convenient snack food avoiding sugar

Healthy Smoothie Ingredients

Smoothies are perfect for breakfast. They also make a refreshing snack or a healthy desert. Smoothies can be made with a variety of fruit or vegetables or combining both. Frozen fruit is easy to use as no washing, pealing, or slicing is needed. A supply of frozen ingredients in the freezer can always be readily available when fresh fruit is not in season.

Frozen Fruit

Cherries
Blueberries
Strawberries
Mixed Berries
Pineapple
Mangoes
es

Fresh Fruit

Bananas
Strawberries
Cherries
Cantaloupe
Raspberries
Peaches   Peach-
Pineapple

Vegetables

Spinach
Kale
Celery
Cauliflower
Zucchini
Carrots

Liquids

Orange Juice
Coconut Milk
Apple Juice
Almond Milk
3% Milk
Pineapple Juice

To make a smoothie place frozen fruit and other ingredients in a blender. If using fresh fruit in place of frozen be sure to add 2 ice cubes and blend until puree is completely smooth.

Healthy Smoothies

The following recipes, make one generous serving unless noted otherwise.

Cindy's Spinach Splash:

1 cup fresh spinach

1 ripe banana

I cup almond milk

3 large frozen strawberries

1/2 cup blueberries

Carol's Lime Cantaloupe

Juice from 1 small lime

2 cups of sliced cantaloupe

1 cup cold water

1/2 tsp. honey

3 ice cubes

Healthy Smoothies (2)

Virginia's Vanilla Mango

1 cup frozen blueberries

1 kiwi sliced

1 cup almond milk

1 cup of chopped mango

Barbara's Blueberry

1 1/2 cups of apple juice

1 chopped banana

1 cup frozen blueberries

3/4 cup plain yogurt

Ava's Peanut Butter Banana

1/2 cup almond milk

1 1/2 T. peanut butter

1 chopped banana

1/4 cup Greek yogurt

3 ice cubes

Healthy Smoothies (3)

Paula's Banana Pineapple

1/4 fresh pineapple peeled, cored and cubed

1 large banana cut into chunks

1 cup pineapple or apple juice

3 ice cubes

Anna's Banana Cherry

1/2 cup frozen cherries

I cup almond milk

1 banana

1 T. vanilla yogurt

Kate's Banana Kale

2 ripe bananas chopped

1/2 cup chopped kale

1/2 cup fresh orange juice

1/2 cup plain yogurt

1/2 T. honey

3 ice cubes

Healthy Smoothies (4)

Alexandria's Banana Brain Booster

2 cups of 3% whole milk

1 banana, slightly over ripe

3 large frozen strawberries

1/2 cup frozen blueberries

Cindy's Coconut Pineapple

1 1/2 cups frozen pineapple chunks

1/4 cup coconut milk

1/4 cup pineapple juice

1/4 cup vanilla yogurt

1 T. unsweetened shredded coconut

Susan's Strawberry Banana

11/2 cups frozen strawberries

1 banana

1 T. orange juice concentrate

1 cup vanilla soy milk

Healthy Smoothies (5)

Berry Banana Cauliflower

1/2 cup frozen cauliflower pieces

1/4 cup mixed berries

1 cup sliced frozen banana

1 cup almond milk

2 tsp. maple syrup

Brenda's Banana Yogurt

1 banana

1/2 cup plain yogurt

1 tsp. honey

1/4 cup pineapple juice

1 cup mixed berries

1 tsp. orange juice

1 tsp. milk

Laughter is a great way
to begin a friendship
and is great way
to discourage dementia.

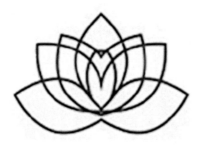

Tool #6

Avoid Isolation

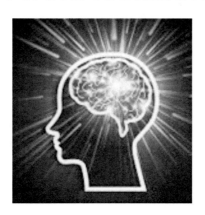

My grandmother taught me that
happiness is both a skill and a
decision. You are responsible
for the outcome.

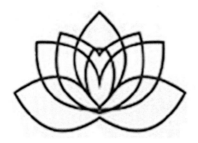

Avoid Isolation (1)

Social interaction is a basic human need and will impact the health and quality of life of older adults. It is a fact that infants who don't receive touching and involvement with others often fail to thrive. American jailers have determined that solitary confinement is a catastrophic brain punishment.

The need for social interaction doesn't change as we age. In fact, it may become even more important to thriving in advanced age than diet or exercise. Loneliness can lead to numerous health issues including dementia. In addition social isolation causes meaningless sensitivity to social threats and potentially harmful thoughts.

Elderly people who are involved, outgoing and gift-giving are usually not as easily stressed and are less likely to develop dementia.

Regardless of how social isolation occurs, the result is that basic needs for authentic intimacy remain. One in three people will die possibly from another disease or heart failure but will have had dementia disorder. It is therefore vital to keep mentally and physically active throughout life and at all costs avoid loneliness and isolation.

Avoid Isolation (2)

Few people look forward to losing their spouse or family member, living alone, to carry on without families or friends to share stories and offer support when problems occur. However, many North Americans are facing this as numbers of seniors pass away and their partners are left alone to grieve. Literally thousands, primarily older women are left alone in various forms of isolation.

It is reported on-line that over 11 million people, 28% of those aged 65 and older are now living alone and the number is growing as the baby boomers reach retirement age. They did not have children or the children have relocated to other cities. There are fewer family members located close by to ensure a parent is provided with frequent visits and invited to social or family events.

Approximately 50% of single elderly women living without an active social life residing in a rental apartment or a retirement residences, make absolutely no effort to participate in community social programs.

Some older people have a disinterest in social involvement. Many, primarily due to years of avoiding social connections, lack confidence. In some cases their partner did not encourage a social lifestyle. Regardless of the cause, the results can be devastating. Loneliness can result in depression and for many the onset of dementia.

Avoid Isolation (3)

Let us consider the mother or father who married young, had 2 to 6 children and did not complete any formal education. They might have spent 30 years without any serious brain challenges or stimulation and without creating cognitive reserves.

They may have raised amazing children, managed a wonderful, loving home, proud parents with an exceptional family. The question is whether their jobs or home responsibilities prevented either of them from building cognitive reserves and therefore leaving them susceptible to dementia, did either of them have an active social life ?

Did either of them have an active brain, play challenging games, enjoyed reading, have a brain stimulating hobby or other challenging brain activities? When one passed, did the remaining spouse expand their world or choose to live in isolation ?

Make New Friends
Later in Life

Securing new friends does take a little effort but the benefits can be amazing, and will certainly enhance a person's life. There is a multitude of community clubs and social groups where you will meet people with similar interests. Building a network of like minded friends can be an interesting adventure, establishing a new friendship that may last for years.

How about "The Red Hat Society" is an international social organization primarily for women over 50 years of age, but is now open to younger ladies. The club is focused on helping women live a full life and adventure. The goal, never, ever being lonely. For the men the "Men's Shed" or a "Legion". Men's Shed originated in Australia now has over 2,200 associate clubs world wide. Most meet weekly. Most members are 65 plus and interested in hobbies, woodworking, computers, cards and fellowship. The local Legion or Veterans club will have a seniors' active auxiliary involved in bowling, a book club, golf, bingo, billiards, shuffleboard and dancing. A great way to meet new friends.

Seniors' Associations are the most active and most popular. Clubs with 200 to 2,000 members offer every possible   activity. Membership fees are usually very reasonable, $35 to $50 a year, with a separate fee for specific activities.

Loneliness

There are approximately 5 million people in North America living alone and about 40% of these often go for 5 to 7 days with little socializing.

Over 50% of people age 75 or older live alone.
Over 25% of older people depend on their television as main social connection.

Loneliness is a complex and usually unpleasant emotional response to isolation. Loneliness typically includes anxious feeling about a lack of connection or communication with other human beings, both in the present and extending into the future. As such loneliness can be felt even when surrounded with other people.

Loneliness has a direct connection to the development of de-mentia. Hundreds of older men and women have slowly drifted into their shells having little or no connection with their families or friends which promotes dementia. This is prevalent even in seniors retirement residences, where it is not uncommon to have a large number of residents living in isolation, seldom leaving their apartments. When dining they tend to avoid discussions with others at their table and quickly return to their apartments after eating.

The bottom line is I have had a

wonderful long life.

I took care of myself, kept busy

and had many great friends.

I am just Betty, I am the same Betty

I have always been, take it or leave it!

.   Betty White

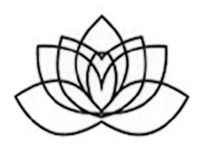

Tool #7

Be A Constant Learner

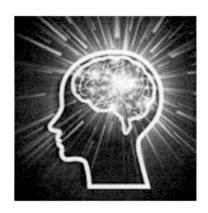

Be a Rainbow in someone
else's cloud.

Maya Angelou

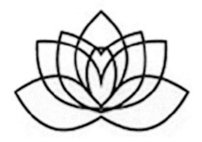

Be a Constant Learner

Both the UK and Finland have discovered that people who continue in education have a lower risk of developing dementia. The brains of over 800 people who had been part of three large ageing studies were examined. Before their deaths they had completed questionnaires about education. Researchers found that more   education makes people better able to cope with changes in the brain associated with dementia.

Over the past decade, dementia patients have consistently supported the concept that proves the longer you continue in education, the lower the risk of dementia. For each additional year of education there could be an 11% decrease in the risk of dementia.

Apparently the level of education associated with risk of dementia varied by years of education. A more consistent relationship with dementia occurred when years of education reflected cognitive capacity. This again suggests that a   lifetime of education will greatly lower the risk of dementia.

Research continues in these countries which is needed to fully understand how education supports the brain and the brain's reserves. But there is little doubt that keeping the brain active and engaged by learning new skills is a powerful tool to avoid dementia.

Lifelong Education

In most cities there are two types of lifelong learning (also called continuing education) opportunities for seniors. You can pay a discounted tuition fee and join younger students in regular credit or non-credit courses, or mingle with other elders in non-credit, mostly daytime, senior specific programs, usually at modest cost.

Here are some other learning suggestions:

Join an advocacy group

Visit the internet which offers hundreds of courses

Watch game shows such as Jeopardy on television

Buy Trivia books

Attend age appropriate acting classes

Take cooking classes

Attend government sessions, join a political party

Study the body and health issues

Take up mentally challenging hobbies

Visit your library on a regular schedule

Join a book club

Assemble a group and pick subjects for discussion

Read about plants and herbs

Consider writing your own trivia book with multiple choice answers based on your favorite subject

Music is the divine way to tell beautiful,
poetic things to the heart.

Pablo Casals

A day without laughter
is a day wasted.

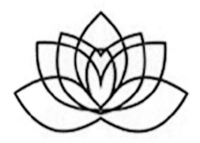

Tool #8

Manage Stress

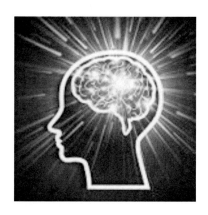

Be tender with the young
compassionate with the aged
considerate of the weak.
Some day in your life
you will be all of the above.

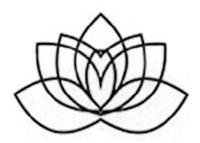

Manage Stress (1)

Stress can be good or bad depending on how much control we believe we have over the outcome. If we think we can manage, then we have less stress.

If we dwell on the threat, the greater our fear and the greater our stress.

Recognize the symptoms of stress:

Headaches

Difficulty getting proper sleep

Leg cramps

Head and neck pain

Poor appetite

Mood swings

Frequent anger

Lack of concentration

.

Manage Stress (2)

Stress and tension are normal reactions to events that threaten us. Stress reduction is an important part of a healthy lifestyle, just like diet and exercise. Stress can occur at any time. The following suggestions will help you learn how to manage stress.

- Recognize the symptoms of stress

- Put problems in perspective

- Regular physical activity such as yoga, meditation and daily exercise

- Clear the mind

- Resolve issues before they become critical

- Limit alcohol, coffee, sugar, fats and tobacco

- Have a restful nights sleep

- Talk with a friend or a counselor

- Accept those things that are beyond your control

Manage Stress (3)

Help others. Volunteer work can be an effective and a satisfying stress reducer.

Read a book, watch a movie, play a game, listen to music or go on a vacation. Have some time that's just for you.

Become physically active. Plant a garden, clip the flowers, start a new project, clean the car, clean the house, sort out the junk.

Ease up on criticism of others, avoid quarrels, learn to compromise.

Stress has a disturbing effect, we can predict the likelihood that a person will become ill based on the number of recent changes in his or her life.

Too much positive change can be just as bad as too much negative change.

Too little work can create almost as much stress as too much work because the brain requires a certain level of stimulation to be properly engaged and functioning.

Slow Progress
Is Better Than
No Progress

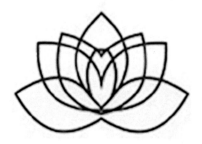

Tool #9
Live a
Happy Life

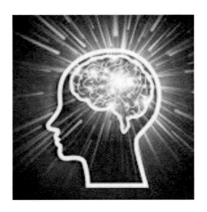

Compassion is a language the deaf
can hear and the blind can see.

Mark Twain

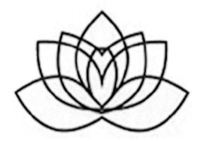

Live a Happy Life (1)

Happiness is the meaning and the purpose of life. Simple joys in life bring real happiness. The following are suggestions to live a happy, satisfying life:

1. Do what you love. If your passion is playing soccer, writing poems, teaching, drawing, art, a hobby, playing golf, make time to do it. You will find when you are doing what you love, you're filled with joy and satisfaction. That is much better than doing things that which dull the brain.

2. Help others. There is nothing, absolutely nothing as rewarding as helping someone else. It makes you feel wonderful.

3. Be thankful, appreciate all the things you have and how blessed you are: a roof over your head, food to eat, a wonderful country, freedom and lasting friendships.

4. Share with others and learn to listen. Share your thoughts with others and listen intently as they share theirs with you.

5. The world loves a person who is a good listener.

6. Smile more. A smile will make you a happier person.

Live a Happy Life (2)

7. Smile in a crowd, in a restaurant, at the bank teller, at your postman, post lady or delivery person. Ask for their name. Smile while talking on the phone.

8. Give gifts. They don't have to be expensive, a card, a poem, a quick note, e-mail, or a magazine. Brighten someone's day and this will brighten yours.

9. Take a walk outdoors, enjoy nature and fresh air.

10. Be yourself. Life is very short, don't waste it. Accept who you are, just be yourself. Have confidence and self satisfaction. Above all keep smiling.

11. Forgive and forget. Holding a grudge will harm you more than the person you're holding a grudge against.

12. Focus on the good things in life.

13. Eliminate negative thinking, Negative thoughts will bring you down. Replace them with positive thoughts.

14. Spend more time with positive people, you will live a happier and more interesting life.

15. People who are happy and positive will likely have better health and a real defense against dementia.

Live a Happy Life (3)

- Interact with family and friends
- Foster strong long term friendships
- Spend time with interesting people
- Be in harmony with a spouse or partner
- Find a new friend and celebrate old friends
- Find a meaningful community commitment

- Have enough savings
- Commit to a volunteer project
- Take an afternoon nap
- Forgive someone
- Make the final payment on a loan
- Be grateful for your position in life

- Have a fun experience with a friend
- Listen to soothing music
- Work on your bucket list
- Achieve a long term goal
- Wake up in the morning with a smile
- Be positive
- Have a hobby
- Have a supply of DVD concerts

Live a Happy Life (4)

Brain Happy Occupations

An on-line fact finding search indicates teachers, lawyers, doctors and accountants are professions which normally protect the brain and avoid dementia.

Numerous web sites indicate employment that involves 'complex social interaction', such as mentoring, negotiating or teaching, are what help to fight against disorders setting into a failing brain.

These discoveries advance the theory that a mentally engaged lifestyle can reduce the harmful effect that abnormal brain changes have on cognitive wellness. These studies do claim this is primarily about the interaction with people, engaging with others on a regular basis. Interaction plays an important role in boosting cognitive reserve.

Being socially active and mentally engaged, in work and personal life, are the keys to keep the mind and memory healthy, alive and anxious to take on new challenges.

Bad things do happen. How one responds to these defines one's character and quality of life. They can choose to sit in perpetual sadness, immobilized by gravity of loss, or can choose to rise above the pain and treasure the most precious gift of all, life itself.

Tool #10

Encourage Laughter

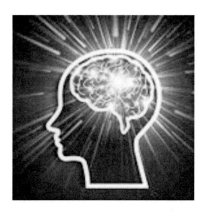

Laughter is the Best Medicine

Yes, it's fun to share a good laugh. But did you know it can actually improve your health?

It's true. Laughter is an amazing medicine. It brings people together in ways that trigger healthy physical and emotional changes to the body. Laughter strengthens the immune system, relieves pain and protects against the damaging effects of stress.

Laughter is the sweetest medicine for the mind and body. Laughter is a powerful antidote to stress, pain and conflict. Nothing works faster or more dependably to bring your mood and body back into balance than a good laugh.

Humor lightens burdens and inspires hope which connects you to others and keeps you grounded, focused and alert. It also helps to release anger and be more forgiving. **Best of all, this priceless medicine is fun, free and easy to use.**

A good laugh relieves physical tension and stress, leaving your muscles relaxed for up to 45 minutes after. Laugher decreases stress and is an important tool in our fight to avoid or reverse dementia.

Laughter protects the heart, improves the function of blood vessels and increases blood flow which helps to protect against heart attacks or strokes. Strokes can result in dementia.

Laughter burns calories. This is not a replacement for the stationary exercise bike or a brisk walk. Laughing for 10 or 15 minutes a day can burn off about 40 calories, a fun way to lose a few pounds.

People who have a positive outlook on life tend to fight memory loss and dementia better than people who tend to be negative. **So smile, laugh and live a longer, healthier and happier life.**

There is only one true super power amongst human beings and that is being funny. People treat you differently if you can help make them laugh.

A Study of Laughter in Norway

Laughter may help you to live longer. In Norway they have determined that people with a strong sense of humor outlive those who don't laugh much. They discovered the difference was particularly notable for those battling dementia and cancer.

Laughter is good medicine

Helps to delay and/or avoid dementia

Reduces anxiety

Laughter is an immune boosting therapy

Lowers stress, anger and sadness

Decreases pain

Relaxes muscles

Helps prevent heart disease

Decreases stress

Improves mood

Decreases blood pressure

Strengthens resilience

Strengthens relationships

Draws you closer to others

Enhances teamwork

Builds lasting friendships

Adds joy and zest to life

Tool #11

Be Musically Inspired

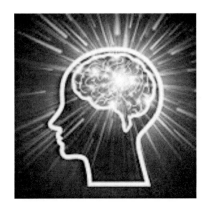

There are four kinds of people in the world:
Those who have been care givers;
Those who currently caregivers;
Those who will be caregivers;
And those who will someday need care givers.

Rosalynn Carter
Former First Lady

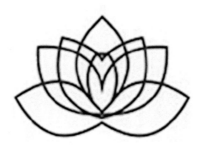

Be Musically Inspired (1)

Music can improve moods and eliminate depression. It can also improve blood flow in ways similar to cholesterol medication and lower stress levels. Music can also relieve pain. How does this happen? Music helps the brain develop memory and a positive mood. Music can boost a person's well-being improve stress related pressures and eliminate a troubled, confused mind. Particularly those who might be experiencing early dementia.

Listening to calm music is a powerful tool for improving overall health. Music with a slow tempo is usually calming while loud annoying music can have the opposite effect.

There is no common music that appeals to everyone. Music that is recognizable can create a more positive response than music which in unfamiliar. Like other things in life, familiarity provides some degree of comfort. Uncommon music can be stressful because it is annoying, stressing the brain. When a person listens to a new piece of music the brain tends to be searching for words and melody. Familiar uplifting music offers healthy great benefits helping to soothe the brain.

Be Musically Inspired (2)

In England the benefits of music are a proven fact with government agencies supporting sing along sessions at seniors retirement homes throughout the country. Certain types of music, especially classical, can boost a person's brain power. Participants typically respond more strongly to live music played by real people. Encouraging seniors' to sing along and dance to the music offers amazing therapy.

Music Unlocks Memories (1)

The power of music, especially singing, to unlock memories and kick start the grey matter is an increasingly key wellness feature. It seems to reach parts of the damaged brain in ways other forms of communication can not.

If you love listening to music, you're in good company. Ronald Reagan said, "If I had my life to live over again, I would have made it a rule to read some poetry or listen to some music each day." Music has amazing benefits and has a direct influence in avoiding or delaying dementia, says Professor John Wainwright, an academic who has made a study of the effect of music in dementia care.

We know that the auditory system of the brain is the first to function at age 16 weeks, which means that you are musically receptive long before anything else. So it's a case of first-in-last - out when it comes to a dementia type breakdown in memory.

Music Unlocks Memories (2)

Many music students throughout the U.K. now regard care home visits as part of their learning experience. Live music is enormously beneficial to those with various forms of dementia as well as to the care givers. It is also helpful and rewarding for the musicians.

Organizations like 'Singing For the Brain', 'Music for Life', 'Lost Chord', and 'Golden Oldies' have made it possible for every care home in England to have access to live musicians. Entertainers have learned how to deal with the special needs of an elderly, memory impaired audience.

Singing For the Brain

'Singing For the Brain' is run by the Alzheimer's / Dementia Society in 30 different locations in England nationwide. It aims to boost confidence, self esteem and quality of life by involving people with dementia in inter-active sing song sessions.

One lady with dementia who didn't know her own name any longer, knew every song in a quiz, sang them all and was on her feet keeping time to the music.

There is a growing verification that music can help to delay early dementia disorder. Memory and awareness are greatly improved by listening and participating in group sessions.

The Power of Music (1)

The human brain is connected to music with long term memory. For those who have symptoms of early dementia, familiar music can often trigger otherwise hidden memories enabling the listener to focus on the present moment and to   regain a revived connection to family and friends. There are many benefits with music intervention which have been studied. These include improved memory, verbal communication and physical activity.

Music is directly linked to the memory. Music can reduce agitation and in turn dementia, lessen anxiety, reduce pain, lower blood pressure, help with sleep and increase cooperation. Music releases dopamine, a 'feel-good transmitter' in the brain.

It is strongly recommend that those who suspect early dementia or even those with advanced dementia purchase a portable music player with earphones, which can be played at any time without disturbing others.

Record the loved one's favorite music on a device that will recall pleasant memories.

The Power of Music (2)

Music response may be dependent upon harmony, tempo, rhythm, melody, timbre, instrumentation etc. Music with a slow, rhythmic tempo can be relaxing. Music with a pattern or that is sedative can be very relaxing and discourage mood swings.

Research has proven that when you listen to music you like, your brain releases dopamine a 'feel-good' neurotransmitter. So the next time you need an emotional boost, listen to your favorite tunes for 15 minutes, That's all it takes to get a natural high!

"Oh, What a Beautiful Morning"

The personality of the listener comes into play as a variable: age, intellect, ethnicity, environment, economy, religion,   education, and other personality factors. If the music is familiar and pleasing it will have a greater effect.

As an example, a seniors retirement residence in Australia provides background music during morning breakfast with songs such as "Oh, What a Beautiful Morning" followed by other popular up-beat oldies. The mood and the general atmosphere is obviously brighter and starts the residents day off with a happier attitude.

The Amazing Benefits of Music

- Music makes you happier
- Music reduces anxiety
- Music raises IQ
- Music improves exercise
- Music lowers stress
- Music helps you sleep better
- Music improves health as we age
- Music reduces pain
- Music improves cognition
- Music discourages over eating
- Music strengthens memory
- Music improves recovery from strokes
- Music helps to delay or avoid dementia
- Music provides comfort
- Music elevates mood while driving

Tool #12

Refresh and Energize

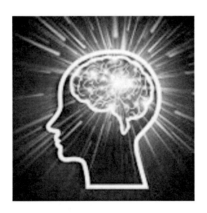

Refresh and Energize
Take Two Painting Classes
and Call Me in the Morning

What if you were ill and instead of, or along with, a doctor wrote you a prescription for a music, dance or painting class?

Doctors in Britain may soon be prescribing such activities for a range of illnesses including **dementia.** In a speech the British Health minister (Matt Hanncock) decried over medication, set out the benefits of social prescribing across the board, from arts to physical exercise to nutritional advice.

Hannock said "Through learning to play instruments, trying conducting and eventually performing as part of an orchestra, nearly 90 per cent of stroke patients felt better physically with fewer dizzy spells, epileptic seizures, less anxiety, improved sleep, improved concentration and memory". He also cited a project which used dance to improve communication and well being.

Doctors in Montreal recently experimented with handing out free museum passes to patients. Studies have shown that exposure to the arts improves the health of older people with **dementia.**

Mayo Clinic is also developing degree programs in medical humanities at its Alix School of Medicine. Such programs are becoming more common across the United States.

Refresh and Energize (1)

Brain Stimulating Projects

Antique Collecting

Art Lessons

Ceramics / Pottery

Astrology

Auto Restoration

Bicycle Repairs

Feed the Birds

Calligraphy

Candle Making

Board or Foster a Pet

Own a Pet

Clock Building

Clock Collecting

Coin Collecting

Computer Coding

Computer Repairs

Cooking / Baking

Cosmetology

Crocheting

Tour Guide

Doll Making

Habitat for Humanity (volunteering)

Meals on Wheels (volunteering)

Refresh and Energize (2)

Brain Stimulating Projects

Design & Make Jewelry

Sewing

Embroidery

Leather Works

Be a Magician, present Magic Shows

Host a Trivia Show

Learn How to Create Stained Glass

Gift Creations

Wood Working

Wood Carving

Dancing (Learn New Steps)

Miniature House Building

Model Airplane Building

Become an Exceptional Soup Chef

Publish Your Own Soup Cook Book

Become a Tin Crafter
Learn computer coding

Brain Stimulating Projects (1)

Create Fantasy Jewelry

Be creative. Design and make decorative gifts and fun, elegant jewelry. Easy to set up at home and invite a friend to work on a project with you.

For more information visit www.sprucecrafts.com

Become an Author, Write a Story

The best way to defeat writers block is to begin writing. Choose a topic that is of interest to you. Your town or city, exciting restaurants, favorite foods, pets, personal interests or choose a current topic.

visit www.thewriterspractise.com

Become a Leather Crafter

You can purchase leather, tools and fittings and learn how to make wallets, a purse, book covers or even a jacket. Painting on leather can create a fabulous gift.

visit www.shastaleather.com

Feed the Birds

Watching a variety of birds visiting your yard is a great pleasure in summer and winter. Put out a filled birdfeeder hanging from a post or a tree which is visible from the comfort of your home. Bird watching will become a daily event. As the seasons change a variety of feathered friends will visit. Feeding birds is a peaceful rewarding experience.

visit The Canadian Wildlife Federation on-line.

Organize a Wizard Card Group

Wizard has been selected as the #1 brain strategy game, excellent for dementia brain wellness. Either 4, 5 or 6 players. Organize a weekly program at a home or club. Our own club currently has 36 members, weekly scores are recorded and prizes are awarded quarterly. We play 3 games each sessions, $1 per player, per game, with 6 players the winning pot is $6. Each player notates $2 to pay for treats. A fun event.

Brain Stimulating Projects (2)

Make Candy

Start making candy at home! Whether you're a novice in the kitchen or an experienced cook try expressing your creativity making candy and surprising friends, family or complete strangers. You will be a very popular person. Go on-line for instructions, select only the best ingredients to ensure a successful and delicious treat. Cut back on the sugar.
visit www.thespruceeats.com

Learn to Crochet

Visit the following web site for a step by step guide which will get you started with basic crochet techniques. When you first begin, the instructions may seem confusing, don't be discouraged it is not that difficult.
visit www.craftey.com

Make Dolls

Go on-line for instructions. Most likely the first doll will not turn out exactly as planned, but you will love it anyway. The joy is on the face of the little girl who knows that you made the doll specifically for her.
visit www.adelepo.com

Adopt a Pet

Pets provide love and fill our need for companionship. My family has had 13 dogs over the years each with it's own different and unique personality. It is a fact that people who own pets have fewer medical issues. While dogs are the first to come to mind, cats are the favorite of millions of people and we have friends who are on their second pet rabbit. If ownership is too much of a commitment you might consider volunteering at your local animal shelter or board pets while the owners are away on vacation.

Brain Stimulating Projects (3)

Play Sudoku to Sharpen Your Brain

Sudoku without question is one of the greatest brain exercise tools that anyone can employ as a defense against dementia.
At first it is frustrating but you will soon be hooked. Sudoku is a game of logic, problem solving and spotting patterns. It is a true Brain Game that helps stimulate cognitive abilities and gives the satisfaction of solving a difficult puzzle.
visit.www.instructables.com

Become a Magician

If you like impressing friends or making a little money at birthday parties, at a local bar or community events you could become a magician. Start learning a few simple tricks and then work your way up to more complex illusions. Start with card tricks, misdirection and coin tricks. Rabbits that appear out of a hat will come later.
Various books and web sites on-line

Tin Crafting

Instead of recycling your tin and aluminum cans turn them into art objects. Create useful objects or amazing gifts. You could make pencil holders, candlesticks, bird feeders, holders for odds and sods, fireplace match holders or let your imagination wander. Have some fun and connect with others selling your new creations at a community fair?

Be a Soup Chef

Soup is one of the simplest foods. Take up the challenge and make soups the old fashioned way. It does take a little more time but the results can produce a healthy delicious meal !

Restful Sleep (1)

The combination of a healthy diet, moderate daily exercise and a night of restful sleep will result in a healthy mind and body.

The direct benefits of a regular sleep routine:

Improved social skills
Enhanced memory
Happy outlook on life
Improved concentration
Sleep rids the brain of toxins
Improved immune system
Weight control
Increased energy
Helps control stress

Suggestions to enhance sleep:

Develop a constant sleep routine. Fall asleep and re-awake at the same time each day.

Limit caffeine.

Avoid a heavy meal and fried foods at dinner time.

Avoid TV and computer media screens 2 hours prior to bed time as blue light emitted will cause sleep disruption.

To fall asleep repeat the words "Go To Sleep' over and over and over. It works, you will quickly fall asleep.

Restful Sleep (2)

Invest in a comfortable bed

Sleep in a cool room

Cover windows

Have a sleep eye mask

Have a warm bath

Listen to calm music

Do a few low impact stretches to relax muscles

Learn to relax. Close your eyes and take deep slow breathes, each breath deeper than the last. Concentrate on your breathing, clearing the mind of other thoughts.

Have a pad of paper and pencil to record any thoughts or if you wake up with some worry-some problems postpone these issues until morning.

There are various theories on napping during the day. A 30 minute nap can be energizing and refreshing, a wonderful opportunity to recharge.

If a person has early stage dementia, a regular nap is a helpful wellness tool but must be combined with brain activities.

I'm always doing that
which I cannot do, in
order that I may learn
how to do it !

Pablo Picasso

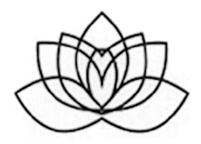

Live Longer

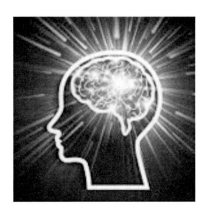

Live Longer

The world population balance is changing dramatically. In 2010 an estimated 524 million people in the world were aged 65 or older, which was 8 percent of the world's population. By 2050, this number is expected to nearly triple to about 1.6 billion representing 17 percent of the world's population.

The remarkable change is being driven by the decline in fertility and improvements in longevity. With fewer children entering the population and people living longer, older people represent an increasing share of the total population.

As an example, in France, during the past 100 years the population aged 65 and older has risen from 4 percent to 20 percent, with similar statistics in most major developed countries including Canada and the United States. In 2018 this caused an uprising in France when Emanuel Macron, the French President, decided to increase the pensions of the senior population. The young people suffering from increased taxes revolted and riots continued for weeks.

Live Longer

Although most babies born in 1900 did not live past age 50, life expectancy at birth now exceeds 83 years. In Japan, the world leader, the average age is now 88 years. More than 60 percent of the improvement in life expectancy starting in 1890 is because children did not die at a birth or at a young age, not because more adults were reaching old age. It wasn't until the 20th century that mortality rates began to decline with the older ages. Research for the more recent periods shows a surprising and continuing improvement in life expectancy. People who live to age 90, 100 and older is becoming more common.

The progressive increase in survival in these oldest age groups was not anticipated by demographers and it now raises questions as to predicting the average future life expectancy. What is the potential length of the human life span? While some experts assume that life expectancy must be approaching an upper limit, data on life expectancy between 1890 and 2007 show a steady increase averaging about 3 additional months of life per year.

In 1870 the country with the highest life expectancy was Sweden, today it is Japan. The oldest old are now the fastest growing part of the world population.

Aging and Living Alone

The percentage of older people living alone is rising in most countries. In some European countries, more than 40 percent of women aged 65 or older live alone. Even in societies with strong traditions of older parents living with children, such as Japan and the Philippines, traditional living arrangements are becoming less common.

In many countries older people prefer to live in their own homes even if it means living alone. However, many of the oldest-old lose their ability to live independently because of limited mobility, safety or forgetfulness. Many require some form of long-term care, which may include home nursing and community care and/or assisted living. The significant costs associated with providing support will be incurred by families as governments struggle with these ever increasing unmanageable costs.

The real challenge in the immediate and coming years for public health and wellness advisors is to educate and encourage the population. Unless the population includes dementia prevention in their lives, over 33 percent will be facing dementia at age 65 to 85, at which time there will be little or no facilities available to care for them.

The World Population is Aging

The world population is aging at an unprecedented rate. By 2040 the percentage of seniors in most countries will double or triple. I have prepared the following somewhat shocking chart illustrating a rapid decline in births and huge growth in numbers of people age 65 to 95 years of age.

	As a percentage of the country's population			
	age 14 and under		age 65 and older	
	1960	2017	current	year 2050
Japan	30%	13%	29%	36%
Canada	34%	16%	21%	34%
United States	31%	19%	16%	32%
United Kingdom	23%	18%	18%	36%
France	26%	18%	20%	39%
Germany	21%	13%	22%	36%
Russia	30%	18%	14%	26%
World	36%	26%	7%	15%

By the year 2050 the total number of people under 20 years of age combined with those over 65 will potentially represent as much as 50% of the world population. This will dramatically increase health costs and place enormous pressure on govern-ment sponsored retirement facilities, hospitals and families.

Reading is important because
you can read, you can learn anything
about anything, about everything about
everything and everything
about anything.

Tomie dePaola

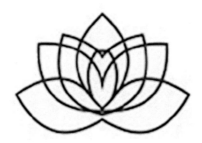

Benefits of Reading (1)

Reading has many benefits and is especially important as we consider the effects for those determined to avoid dementia. Here are 15 reasons to be a constant reader.

1. Mental Stimulation

Your brain requires exercise to keep it strong and healthy, just like the muscles in your body. Reading has been found to enhance connectivity in the brain. A decline in memory and brain function is a side effect of aging, but regular reading may help slow the process. **Keeping your brain active and engaged can slow the progress of dementia.**

2. Stress Relief

When reading you must focus on the characters and the plot of the book. The gateway into the literary world allows you to distance yourself from the stress of everyday life, putting your mind and body at ease. Losing yourself in a great story can be a perfect remedy for stress.

3. Restful Sleep

Sometimes it is hard to fall asleep when your mind is racing and busy worrying about a variety of things. Reading, even if just for ten minutes, can help you push aside whatever was keeping you awake. Bright lights from electronic devices can signal your brain that it is time to wake up. Reading under a dim light can be more beneficial when trying to fall asleep. Make sure your book

Benefits of Reading (2)

is not a page turner, one that you can't possibly put down. A book of poetry or inspiring quotations may be a better choice. A biography might also be an excellent choice.

4. Education

Education is not cheap. Classes, seminars and educational software are just a few of the ways that you can pay to learn. However, reading books from the library is free! If you find a topic that you would like to learn more about, there is a high probability you will find a book in your library that will expand your interest and your education on this subject.

5. Improves Memory

A book has many different components such as the plot, characters, dialogue and settings. Reading requires you to use your memory. Exercising your brain in mentally challenging ways can lead to a slower rate of **decline in memory and help to avoid dementia.** Regular mental exercise through reading can strengthen the network of the brain which helps your mind become more receptive to memory retention.

Benefits of Reading (3)

6. Increases Empathy

Empathy is the ability to understand and share the feelings of another. When we read a fictional story, well-written, we learn to relate to one or two characters in the book. They come to life for us as we read. We feel their pain as they go through certain experiences. Reading helps us to better understand the people around us by putting ourselves in their shoes.

7. Improves Concentration

In today's world our attention is often drawn in a million different directions. When reading you are concentrating on one thing. By doing so, you are training your mind to avoid distractions. This ability can help when performing other tasks that require your attention and concentration.

8. Entertainment

Reading is less expensive than going to the movies or other forms of entertainment. Reading is free at your local library and new books are constantly added. You might be on the wait list for a new highly publicized title, but it will be worth the wait. Books can transport you to different parts of world, all without having to pay airfare.

Benefits of Reading (4)

9. Vocabulary Expansion

The more you read, the more words you are exposed to. Did you know there are over 3,000 new words added to the Oxford Dictionary each year? Being well-spoken and articulate can help increase job performance, self esteem and make you a more interesting person. Exposure to well-written work can also have a huge impact on your writing skills. You may notice that the language in children's books is likely to be more sophisticated than your average conversation.

10. Reading can improve the analytical and reasoning power of seniors as well those with dementia who need to solve problems.

11. Delay Dementia

Challenging brain activities such as reading will build a reserve of brain cell connections and **may help delay or reverse the symptoms of dementia.**

12. Reading Helps Prevent Depression

Depression causes hopelessness, and people with dementia may just give up. It is important that those with dementia symptoms learn to focus on happiness and future potential.

Benefits of Reading (5)

13. Reading is Relaxing

It may be hard to understand but we have reason to believe that reading can be more relaxing than listening to your favorite music, going for a walk or even having that casual cup of tea or coffee.

14. Reading Builds a Critical Mind

The more you read, the more interesting information will be absorbed by your memory. To read and understand what you read your brain must learn to focus.

15. Book Clubs

A great way to meet new people and find enjoyment in reading is to join a Book Club. Different points of view will result in a good discussion of the book and the characters will contribute to your knowledge and appreciation of different cultures, lifestyles and history. Many people read the same genre of books and may not realize how much they would enjoy a different type of book based on a different subject, until they are introduced to new titles by the reading group. A Book Club gathering will provide an enjoyable addition to your social life.

Benefits of Reading (6)

By reading fiction, non fiction, poetry or prose for as little as 30 minutes a day over a lifetime, the brain cells are kept active and receptive to learning and acquiring knowledge. The merits of reading are obvious.

It is a proven fact children who are read to by their parents, starting at six months and throughout their childhood will develop good reading habits that will continue into adulthood. As adults they will have strong literacy skills, score higher in intelligence tests and will have more success in their private and professional lives.

When practiced over a lifetime, those reading and language skills will support brain function which **may guard against dementia.**

Benefits of Reading (7)

Unlike skimming a page of headlines, reading a book forces your brain to think critically and make connections from one chapter to another and to the outside world. When you make connections, so does the brain, literally forging new pathways between regions in all four lobes and both hemispheres of the brain.

Over time, these neural networks can promote thinking more quickly and may provide a greater defense against the worst effects of dementia.

Reading books, especially fiction, has been shown to increase empathy and emotional intelligence. In fact reading anything, including newspapers and magazines, that fills your mind and exposes you to new words, phrases, and facts will provide mental benefits. A large vocabulary will lead to a more resilient mind by fueling cognitive reserve.

Cognitive reserve is the ability of the brain to adapt to damage, just as your blood will clot to cover a cut on your knee. **Cognitive reserve helps your brain cells find new mental   pathways around areas damaged by stroke, dementia and other forms of brain decay.**

Benefits of Reading (8)

So now we should all know we must build up our cognitive reserve. The good news is the vocabulary is resistant to aging. A strong cognitive reserve will significantly delay mental decline. New words and meanings are powerful tools in expanding our vocabulary and social skills while building a healthier brain.

Suggested Books

Tuesdays with Moray
Mitch Albom

Thank You for Being Late
Thomas L. Friedman

A Dog's Way Home
W. Bruce Cameron

Becoming
Michelle Obama

Angela's Ashes
Frank McCourt

The Alice Network
Kate Quinn

Suggested Books

The Girl on the Train
Paula Hawkins

The Everything Store
Brad Stone

Great Expectations
Charles Dickens

Jane Fonda
Patricia Bosworth

Winter of the World
Ken Follett

Fall of the Giants
Ken Follett

The Blue Book
Grammar and Punctuation
Jane Straus

The Runaway Jury
John Grisham

The greatest miracle on earth is
the mind and the human body.
The doctors of the future will
give no medicines, but will interest
his or her patients in the care of
mind and body, in diet, nutrition
and in the causes and prevention
of disease.

Thomas Edison

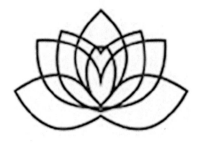

Young Dementia UK (1)

Young Dementia Network is a movement, which originated in England, of people committed to improving the lives of those affected by young onset dementia.

Dementia is considered 'young onset' when it affects people under 65 years of age. It is also referred to as 'early onset' or 'working age' dementia. However, this is an arbitrary age distinction which is becoming less relevant as increased services are realigned to focus on the person and the impact of the condition, not the age.

Dementia a degeneration of the brain that causes a progressive decline in people's ability to think, reason, communicate has been associated with the older generation (65 plus). **However, it is also affecting an increasing number of people in their 40's and 50's.** Their personality, behavior and mood is affected at their place of employment. Everyone's experience of dementia is unique and the progression of the condition varies.

Dementia that affects younger people can be rare and difficult to recognize. People may also be reluctant to accept that anything is wrong when they are otherwise healthy and may put off visiting a doctor.

Although younger people experience similar symptoms to older people, the impact on their lives is significantly different. Younger people are more likely to be still working when they are diagnosed.

Young Dementia UK (2)

Many will have significant financial commitments including a mortgage on their home. They usually have children to care for and possibly dependent parents needing assistance.

Dementia is a life changing condition to have at any age, but when you are young and believe you have a long full life ahead it is most difficult to accept.

Young Dementia UK is currently celebrating 20 years of helping people. Their web site www.youngdementiauk.org provides a host of valuable information including resources, types of dementia in younger people, treatments and therapies, research, family stories, and network connections.

Their web site estimates there are over 42,000 people in the U.K. who have been diagnosed with young onset dementia. This represent around 5% of the 850,000 people with dementia in the U.K. The actual figure could be higher because of the difficulties of diagnosing younger adults, in fact it may be closer to 6% to 9% of young people.

Visit their web site

wwwyoungdementiauk.org

Dementia Stories

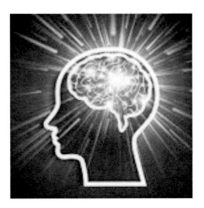

The following dementia stories have been
included to help recognize dementia symptoms
and the related hardships caused by this
dreaded disorder.

Harriet Marshall's Story

My name is Harriett Marshall, I have had an interesting life supporting my husband living on various Canadian military bases around the world. He was a technical advisor, involved in communications for over 22 years.

Unfortunately I am basically a shy person and find I am awkward when it comes to meeting new people. This is a definite liability when you are constantly relocating from city to city. My primary entertainment was reading murder mystery novels.

Things came to a head one day when I suddenly realized I could not remember where I was, what city and what country. It was frightening. Fortunately we were living in a home on a military base. I waited for my husband to come home and shared my problem with him. At first Jim assumed I had a temporary lapse in memory.

But then a week later they found me wandering in a local shopping center which had closed an hour earlier. They called the base medical center who sent medical personnel to pick me up and then contacted Jim. This was the beginning of a series of very disturbing events happening over the next 3 months.

Harriet Marshall's Story (2)

The medical staff in the military had never experienced dementia. It was for older people, not young soldiers and their wives especially when I was age 48, it did not seem possible. It must be something else affecting my memory, possibly I had a stroke without knowing?

Life was becoming very difficult, even forgetting to call my mother back home in Suffield, Canada forgetting what day it was, forgetting to lock the door when I went out, a series of symptoms which we discovered were all related to dementia. Jim requested a relocation back home to Suffield.

Back home I attended a workshop created specifically to help seniors in early stages of dementia. The workshop offered a wide range of assistance and explained the importance of a socially connected life and continuous brain exercises.

I developed a full new life, I met new friends, joined a book club, practiced regular brain memory and physical exercises. I also joined a fun cooking class where we make brain healthy meals. Three years have now passed. Jim and I have studied dementia and memory loss and have made a commitment to work together to defeat this dreaded brain disorder.

Angie's Story

It was in 2012 when I was diagnosed with early onset dementia. I had earlier suspicions that things were not right and decided to work only part time in the florist shop where I had been employed for some 32 years. It is true I did enjoy working at the shop, but I was age 63, had never been married and had for the most part lived a lonely life with almost no outside interests other than television.

It started with my becoming confused with floral arrangements, the customers and delivery schedules. Thankfully the owner of the shop was a friend who was very patient and understanding. It slowly got more serious, I was not recognizing regular customers and the memory difficulties became more troublesome. I then decided I had to give up my job and to move into The Oakwood Manor, a dementia retirement residence.

The social wellness director at the residence encouraged me to purchase a computer to create a reminder calendar and join the 'Become an Author', a fun group. This included some volunteer coaches who provided valued guidance. Initially about a subject we might be interested in, or writing about our own life history. Through this program I discovered I had some unknown talents and met a number of special people who have become my close friends.

Angie's Story (2)

Next I discovered I was able to use my computer to expand my knowledge in a variety of new and very interesting subjects. But most importantly I began attending 'Wake Up the Brain' mini workshops which were presented twice each week in the residence theatre. The presentations described dementia and how with a determined effort one could improve on memory loss and live a less fearful life. We then participated in challenging memory games based on a variety of images and number calculations. All of which encourages brain awareness and stimulation.

I find it hard to read, but I do enjoy audio books and simple brain games on my computer. I now understand that too much television is harmful for the brain, so I make an effort to play card and board games with the others in the social room.

We are blessed with a residence tour bus. We have been to several concerts, the zoo and even a trip to a casino every so often.

Yes, my life has definitely changed for the better. I have occasional memory loss, but I am confident that I am in the right place with people who do care.

Lois and Steven's Story

My name is Steven, I am a retired golf club manager and a suffering dementia love lost husband. This complicated disease has changed my life in so many ways. My wife Lois was a beautiful, wonderful person until one day it all changed. Slowly at first and then suddenly dementia took complete control of my Lois, the woman I love.

Lois had always managed our home, cared for our four children, cooked the meals called the plumber when he was needed, she was amazing. Then one day she was coming home from a dental appointment, about 20 miles from home and she got lost, couldn't find her way home. The police called to say she was found in her car crying. A thoughtful person seeing her had thankfully called the police.

Lois was 65 when we started the diagnosis, it was determined she had phase one dementia and month by month would sink first to phase two and then stage three. It was so sad, I have lost the love of my life, she has disappeared. She is now in a retirement center. At first she often did not recognize me or our adult children. At the center they introduced Lois to a new program based on dementia reversal. Each day she attends a brain   stimulation session, some days memory games, or dance routines,

Lois and Steven's Story (2)

presentations, or a sing along. She is encouraged to participate in regular memory and exercise programs provided by a wellness coordinator at the center.

We are attempting to be positive, her speech is slowly improving, she is encouraged to participate in all the social programs and has met some new friends.

It is very difficult to accept that she will not fully recover from this terrible brain disorder. We must all spend time with her practicing the brain programs. I only wish we had been more aware of dementia when we were younger and included brain wellness dementia prevention programs in our everyday lives back then.

Currently we are working on a historical book centered on Lois's life. The book includes photos, letters, school report cards, newspaper clippings, letters from family and friends all dating back to her younger days. Lois is encouraged to write or dictate a short story or comments for each page of the book which is helping to re-energize and stabilize her memory. This is a fun interesting project which I hope will slowly reverse dementia and will bring her back to me.

Doug and Nancy's Story (1)

Doug

One of my first problems was remembering names of members I would meet at my favorite senior's club. I had always had friends on-line exchanging jokes but I was having trouble with spelling, always getting the letters backwards. When talking I was forgetting the correct word I needed to complete a story or express my thoughts.

My doctor did a thorough examination and suggested I had early stages of dementia. There were drugs he could prescribe but would suggest I first examine my day to day routine, taking steps to sharpen my brain. After review we determined that I had become lazy in both mental and body activities. I had quit my weekly bridge club, was no longer playing golf, and was not a regular reader, which had been one of my favorite activities during almost my entire life.

I was semi-retired, then my employer asked me to leave, so I lost the one activity that had kept my brain working. My doctor said, based on his examination that if I didn't get my brain busy I would likely deteriorate to stage two and then stage three and ultimately would be unable to function.

Doug and Nancy's Story (2)

Nancy

I almost didn't believe this could happen. It shattered my life, a young husband, age 63, with plans to retire and travel together. All our plans and hopes for the future suddenly gone. We have been fortunate the Dementia Society offers real support.

Doug's support worker comes twice a week for mini workshops for both Doug and myself. She takes him for walks and cycling. She goes with him to the seniors' center to make sure he is socially active. She has provided diet information, encouraged drinking wine instead of hard liquor, plus becoming active again doing those things he formerly enjoyed.

The Dementia Society has provided a dementia guide which provides tips on brain health and activities to delay or prevent dementia. We hope that with the proper measures we can live a normal life again.

Helen and Larry's Story (1)

The psychologist arranged for Larry to see a psychiatrist who determined Larry had early stage onset dementia but would probably advance to stage two quite rapidly. I was stunned, Larry was only 58 years of age.

An Opportunity

Suddenly we were offered an opportunity to participate in workshops created for people with dementia. We agreed to participate and quickly realized these were enjoyable, and educational. I slowly noticed a change in my Larry. Then another amazing event, they asked if anyone would be interested in an 'Action on Dementia Group' a committee. I shouted out "Larry will do it", Larry was surprised at my quick response but he agreed to participate.

Larry began attending the committee meetings and it soon became clear that he was regaining his confidence. He now had a purpose in life and his enthusiasm was obvious. He was working twice a week with a group that helps others with memory challenges. He was then encouraged to give talks to medical staff and volunteers about living with dementia.

Helen and Larry's Story (2)

Next came our nephew who helped Larry create a video slide show presentation. Then Larry was introduced on a community TV show and was awarded a "Positive Care" award. Larry was bursting with pride. All through these exceptional changes, the 'Action' program had taught both of us the keys and importance of the brain exercises, interest in new opportunities, proper sleep, daily exercise, nutrition, humor, music and removing stress from our lives.

Don't get me wrong, life is not easy living with Larry and dementia. He can still be troublesome and will argue, when it isn't necessary. On these occasions I just walk away and when I return he is usually back to normal. He just had a memory lapse. Larry may never be the same as he was back then, but he is a lot better than he would have been without the 'Action' program and we are learning how to slow and prevent this dreaded disorder from totally disrupting Larry's brain.

Brenda Swanson's
My Lifestyle Commitment
To Avoid Dementia

I make a constant effort to socialize

I make every effort to challenge my brain

I am committed to a daily exercise program

I walk up the stairs instead of using the elevator

I park a distance from the shops and enjoy the walk

I make every effort to include humor in my life

I take part in challenging brain games

I participate in educational programs

I do not smoke

I drink alcohol in moderation or not at all

I avoid sugars and salts and other harmful foods

I eat fruits & vegetables on a regular basis

I listen to my favorite stimulating music daily

I make an effort to build new friendships

I frequently give gifts to friends and neighbors

Early Stages of Dementia

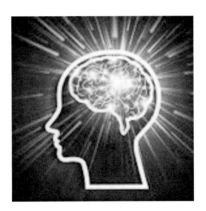

Where there is a will, there is
a way. If there is a chance in a
million that you can do something,
anything, to keep what you want from
ending, do it. Pry the door open, or if
need be, wedge your foot in that door
and keep it open.

Pauline Kael

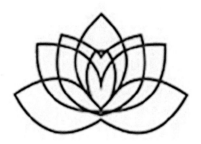

Early Stages of Dementia (1)

In the early stages of a dementia diagnosis the uncertainty of the future can be confusing and somewhat terrifying. In fact as many as 25% of those that receive this diagnosis can return to a normal life within 12 months. It is therefore important that the person remain as active and busy as possible. During the year re-visit the doctor on a regular basis to determine if the symptoms have progressed or disappeared.

Immediately contact your local dementia center to inquire about current programs. Encourage the individual begin 'The 12 Point Tool Box Program' provided in this publication

Remember the person not the dementia. Each person with early dementia will have different symptoms and will respond differently. It is important to focus on the loved one's individual needs, including their history, family, favorite activities, day to day exercises and new events.

Have the loved one tell stories they remember from their childhood. Have a note book to write it all down. Ask them to read these stories to visiting friends or relatives. The person with early dementia needs to feel wanted and looked after because isolation is extremely dangerous.

Early Stages of Dementia (2)

Build a ring binder titled 'My Life' with the person's name printed in large bold type label. Collect as many family photos as possible. Ask the person questions about who, why, where and when related to the photos. Ask questions and offer clues to recharge the person's memory.

Create a slide show of family photos on a computer or other device. Play trivia games with questions related to the photos, or, find old newspapers which report on past major events. Collect stories and images, build an historical slide presentation. Make it a fun, interesting project which can be shared with family and friends. Buy books which illustrate by-gone days in your city or town.

When talking to the person speak calmly and directly. Explain what is happening, encourage them to be involved in the decision making process. Never talk about them when they are close by and can hear your discussion.

Encourage regular activity, being active helps to delay or reverse dementia. Being active and involved in family affairs and events gives the person a sense of purpose.

Early Stages of Dementia (3)

Reduce Frustration

Seniors' who have early dementia might become agitated once simple tasks become more difficult or nearly impossible for them to navigate. They might feel they are always being told what to do by their caregiver or partner.

Boredom and loneliness can be reduced by creating games and activities that stimulate their minds. Establish routines that improve their self confidence. If your senior has difficulty getting involved in conversations, or has a limited attention span, help them to pick activities they can manage.

If the symptoms progress use photos or other visual images to provide instructions for bathroom reminders, directions for brushing teeth, dressing or making a snack.

Early Stages of Dementia (4)

Place photos of family and friends with names placed around the house.

Have photos of family who have past away as a reminder of family history.

Encourage the loved one to participate in preparing a simple meal.

Encourage the loved one to participate in laundry and folding towels and sheets.

Compliment them on work well done.

Prepare an oversized wall calendar to show important dates.

Provide easy-on and off Velcro footwear.

Play regular trivia with multiple choice somewhat easy answers.

Encourage brain exercises as provided in this publication.

Encourage a daily exercise routine.

Include the loved one in family discussions and decisions.

It is important for caregivers to create a safe environment for both the loved one and the entire family. Create a safe home where the loved one can live a normal life doing regular activities safely.

Early Stages of Dementia (5)

Remove clutter, dangerous furniture placement, TV tables, foot stools, fans, rugs that may become rumpled, anything that may cause a person to trip or fall.

Have hand grip bars or rails firmly attached in key areas, have locks installed on the door to the basement, garage door, kitchen cabinets containing knives, kettles, coffee devices, electric appliances or other items that could be dangerous.

Purchase small appliances that shut off automatically.
Install fire and carbon monoxide warning devices.
Create large signs to warn everyone to be attuned to safety.

Be sure the loved one always carries personal information which includes their name, phone number, home address and emergency contact person. Make it oversized with extra large bold print.

Believe in Yourself
and
You'll Be
UNSTOPPABLE

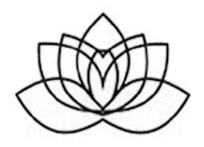

World Review

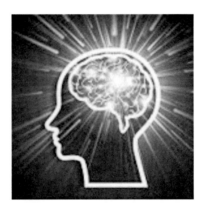

My mission in life is not merely
to survive, but to thrive; and to do
so with some passion, some compassion,
some humor and some style.
Maya Angelou

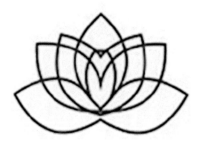

Dementia - World Report 2018

1,   The number of people living with dementia worldwide is currently estimated at 55 million and is projected to increase to 75 million by 2030 and to145 million by 2050.

2. The number of people with dementia who live in low to middle income countries is approximately 30 million.

3. The number of new cases each year is approximately 9.9 million and growing rapidly.

4. The current estimated worldwide costs are $818 billion per year.

5. Caring for dementia patients is an overwhelming challenge for the family, the care giver and the government.

6. Those stricken with dementia can live for 20 to 25 years making this illness the longest and most costly of any of the commonly recognized health issues. Providing a quality of life for a loved one will stretch a families patience and finances possibly for years.

7. In many countries people with dementia and their families are often discriminated against, primarily because there is no cure and no hope for recovery. Compassion is desperately needed.

8. In some countries due to the growing and never ending costs and no known cure, governments are finding it difficult to finance new facilities for dementia patients.

9. Countries must make dementia a priority. More people will die from dementia than cancer and heart disease combined. The world wide cost of dementia care is now greater than cancer and heart disease combined.

10. Government health agencies must encourage and fund seminars and workshops educating those in their younger years to include a dementia prevention wellness program in their daily lives. Also prompting doctors and nurses to encourage their patients to be brain healthy.

The following pages are based on our research. These are many world countries struggling with an ever increasing dementia health problems and related costs. Due to the rapid growth dementia the challenges are ever changing.

Dementia by Country
A Growing World Crisis

Country	Population	Dementia	Percentage
Japan	127 million	4.6 million	3.6
China	1.3 billion	36 million	2.7
South Africa	56 million	1.4 million	2.5
Italy	59 million	1.29 million	2.1
Germany	81 million	1.57 million	1.92
France	63 million	1.1 million	1.85
Canada	36 million	564,000	1.8
Belgium	10.9 million	191,000	1.77
Greece	11.5 million	201,000	1.77
U.S.A.	325 million	5.7 million	1.75
Spain	46 million	818,000	1.75
Australia	25 million	436,000	1.74
Austria	8.4 million	145,000	1.73
Switzerland	7.7 million	133,000	1.72
Finland	5 million	92,200	1.71
Norway	4.9 million	79,000	1.61
Croatia	4.4 million	67,000	1.53
Netherlands	16 million	245,000	1.47
Sweden	9 million	133,000	1.47
Lithuania	3.2 million	67,000	1.44
U.K.	62 million	850,000	1.37
Poland	38 million	501,000	1.31
Ireland	4.6 million	49,000	1.08

In most countries the number of people with dementia is expected to double by 2030 and triple by 2040.

Finland

Finland is experiencing high rates of dementia and has developed continuing programs with the goal of preventing or eliminating dementia.

They tested 1,260 volunteers, aged 60 to 77 at the beginning of the study and then two years later. Those who exercised, changed their diet, made an effort to socialize and did regular memory training did significantly better on the memory tests two years later.

Just two years of exercising, eating healthier foods and practicing brain training boosted their memory function and put them on a path to dementia prevention. The study provides hints at what can be done using common sense tools.

Other studies have shown that people who are socially engaged are less likely to develop memory loss. Still others have shown that keeping the brain active with puzzles or games can help retain a healthy brain. A new brain game industry is evolving in the Scandinavian countries.

Finland has reported considerable success with these programs.

United Kingdom Report
'The Power to Defeat Dementia'

Dementia affects over 850,000 people in the U.K., and currently 706,000 family caregivers. Dementia costs the economy of the U.K. approximately 30 billion U.S. dollars each year and growing. The U.K. currently has the world's most progressive active dementia social and research programs.

Dementia is a progressive and ultimately fatal condition. Over time symptoms grow worse and in later stages people require 24 hour care, by which time they may be unable to communicate and will be experiencing acute psychiatric symptoms.

Current treatments provide modest help with symptoms, but for a limited time and only for only a small percentage of patients. We need treatments that prevent, slow or halt the dementia disorder progression.

The analysis shows that the number of people with dementia in the U.K. are set to grow rapidly over the next 36 years from about 850,000 today to 1,133,000 in 2025 and 2,014,000 by 2050.

U.K. Health report - There is currently no medical solution to prevent dementia. The best evidence is that a healthy lifestyle with an emphasis on brain wellness can help to lower the risk.

Dementia in Canada

More than 564,000 Canadians are currently living with dementia.

As of 2018 the number of Canadians affected directly or indirectly by the dementia disorder is 937,000 and increasing month by month.

Currently 65% of those diagnosed with dementia over the age of 65 are women.

In the year 2018, the number of **Canadians under the age of 65 living with dementia was 16,000.**

It is projected that there will be 60,000 or more new cases of dementia diagnosed every year ongoing.

In Canada there are currently 56,000 patients with dementia being cared for in hospitals even though **this is not an ideal location for those with dementia care.**

They estimate there will be 1.1 million Canadians living with dementia by the year 2032.

The Canadian Federal Government provides financial support for Alzheimer's / Dementia in most major cities across Canada. There is a growing need for mid-life dementia prevention awareness and education.

Dementia in the United States

The number of Americans currently living with dementia is estimated to be 5.9 million. One in 20 Americans age 65 and older (20%) will suffer and probably die with dementia.

Experts project that the number of Americans living with dementia will triple in the next 30 years, over 15 to 25 million will have the mind robbing disorder by the year 2040. It is becoming the leading cause of death in the United States, the total cost being greater than cancer and heart disease combined.

More recent studies suggest that within the next 5 to 7 years dementia will be involved in the deaths of as many as 500,000 people. These are people who will have struggled with this lingering brain disorder for 20 years or more. The costs to the heath system and the patients immediate families will be simply unmanageable.

There is no medical cure and treatments are very ineffective. Doctors are prescribing medications which have little effect on preventing dementia. It is simply a tsunami disorder, especially for the very poor. Doctors are being criticized for prescribing drugs which have no known dementia benefits.

There is a growing need for mid-life dementia awareness and public information.

Dementia in Australia

Australia's population as of January 2019 was 24.7 million.

Dementia is the second highest cause of death of Australians contributing to 5.4% of deaths of men and 10.6% of women in the year 2018.

In 2016 dementia became the leading cause of death among Australian females, surpassing heart disease which has been the leading cause of death of both males and females for the past 100 years.

An average of 36 Australians die each day where dementia is the underlying cause of death. Of the 13,126 people that lost their lives due to dementia, 8,447 were women.

In 2018 there was an estimated 436,000 Australians living with dementia. Without a medical breakthrough, the number of people with dementia is expected to increase to 590,000 by 2028 and over 1 million by 2058.

Currently in Australia 250 people are joining the dementia population each day. **There are over 26,000 people with younger onset dementia, this number will likely rise to 30,000 by the year 2025.**

Dementia in Japan

The life expectancy in Japan is now higher than in any other world country. The number of people now aged 65 and over is in excess of 25% of the total population. Japan's life expectancy is expected to increase to 91 by the year 2030. This is a level of super aging that no world country has ever experienced.

As Japan's population is becoming older it is losing its youth. The percentage of children under 15 years of age has been reduced to 14% of the entire population and is expected to decline even further. More and more women are less interested in marriage and having a family, they want higher education independence and their own income.

In the 20th century Japan's population grew rapidly as the country industrialized. But, in the 1980's the population growth slowed and peaked in 2005. It is now in decline resulting in an imbalance of seniors verses number of children being born. Japan is heading towards a period of enormous costs related to caring for an **ever increasing number of elder Japanese dementia patients needing constant care** .

By the year 2030 approximately 7.3 million (5.7% of the population) will be suffering with dementia based on estimates from the Japanese Health Ministry.

Dementia in Germany

Based the most recent information (year 2012) there were 1,572,104 people suffering with dementia. This represented 1.92% of the total population of 81,990,000. This was somewhat higher than the average of the European Union (1.55%).

The following table shows the estimated number by age.

Age Group	Men	Women	Total
30 - 59	28,656	15,745	44,401
64 - 64	4,740	22,149	26,889
65 - 69	37,007	30,784	67,792
70 - 74	70,514	96,980	167,494
75 - 79	113,093	156,392	269,485
80 - 84	128,627	228,221	356,848
85 - 89	93,540	285,604	379,143
90 - 94	34,516	176,903	211,419
95 +	6,443	42,190	48,663
Total	517,136	1,054,968	1,572,104

Similar dementia information for most European countries can be found on the web site alzheimers-europe.org

Dementia in France

Work has begun on France's first 'Alzheimer's Dementia Village' where patients will be given the free rein without direct supervision in a purpose-built medieval-style citadel designed to increase their freedom and reduce anxiety.

Residents of the village in Dax, southwestern France, will be able to shop in a small supermarket, go to the hairdressers, local brasserie, library, gym and a small farm like area to grow   vegetables and flowers.

They will live in small shared houses designed to reflect their personal tastes and in four districts reminiscent of the south western French region which is between forests and the seashore.

The inhabitants are all men and women suffering from dementia. Allowing them to live in an almost normal village helps patients participate in a social life. Its proponents say this lifestyle is a happier environment when compared to traditional nursing homes. Residents are more active, require less brain deadening medication, they are quite simply happier.

Researchers will conduct a comparative study ongoing with traditional nursing homes and examine the impact of new therapeutic approaches on patients, caregivers and medical staff.

Dementia in France

Based the most recent information (year 2012) there were 1,174,956 people suffering with dementia. This represented 1.85% of the total population of 63,457,777. This was somewhat higher than the average of the European Union (1.55%).

The following table shows the estimated number by age.

Age Group	Men	Women	Total
30 - 59	19,740	11,368	31,108
64 - 64	3,869	18,585	22,254
65 - 69	25,591	21,861	47,811
70 - 74	33,873	47,147	80,930
75 - 79	64,953	94,912	159,865
80 - 84	98,525	178,698	277,274
85 - 89	82,948	228,798	311,746
90 - 94	39,487	152,321	191,808
95 +	6,587	45,424	52,010
Total	375,843	799,113	1,174,956

Similar dementia information for most European countries can be found on the web site alzheimers-europe.org

Dementia in China

China has the largest world population, 1.3 billion people. The number of people living with dementia has shown a steady increase year after year. China now has the largest dementia population. The total number of people with dementia is projected to reach 44 million by 2020 and 48 million by 2030. The total combining Dementia and Alzheimer's disease will be a staggering 75 million by 2030. There were 5 million in 2010.

Given the rapid growth of elderly people in China, dementia is expected to create extreme challenges to the National Health Care system and to the sustainable development of the country's economy. China had a surge in births in the 1950s to 1960s which was followed by plummeting birth rates in the 1970s. China is facing a huge aging imbalance.

Dementia is more common in rural areas than in suburban settings. Yang Honggjie a doctor at the Shanghai Neuromedical Center said dementia brain disorders and Alzheimer's disease could not be cured and there is no effective medicine to treat it. One important treatment to delay the patients' deterioration was to have other people keep them company, help them read, have interesting conversations, play games and build puzzles. A simple chat can do wonders.

In China they predict one third of those who reach age 85 will have dementia and need housing and care. The government is having great difficulty anticipating substantial unmanageable future costs.

Dementia in Russia

The population of greater Russia in 2018 was 146 million. Russia's birth rate is higher than most European countries (13.3 births per 1,000 people compared to the European Union average of 10.1 per 1,000).

Informal sources suggest there are 1.5 million Russians living with dementia. It is estimated 10% of people over 65 years of age and 33% of those 85 or older will have dementia. Life expectancy of those with dementia is 10 to 15 years.

Russian reports indicate dementia is destroying patients lives as well as the lives of immediate relatives and caregivers. Government bulletins suggest that in time relatives begin to recognize the dementia relative is turning into an unmanageable person who may be abusive, may act as a child, who does not recognize family and friends and frequently does not remember happenings from the recent past.

When Russian scientists started researching dementia they identified many factors that slow dementia disorders, including the psychological. For instance, lifestyle, physical activity, enriched environment, cognitive exercises, hobbies, level of education. They indicated all provide important dementia defensive undertakings.

Brain Exercises

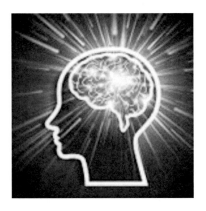

Brain Exercises

Puzzle #1

Select the word that is different

A. Painting

B. Poem

C. Novel

D. Sculpture

E. Flower

F. Embroidery

Puzzle #2

Select the word that is different

G. Pigeon

H. Duck

I. Sparrow

J. Penguin

K. Goose

L. Pelican

See page #205 for answers

Brain Exercises

Puzzle #3

Select the word that is different

A. Frog

B. Swan

C. Beaver

D. Crab

E. Porcupine

F. Duck

Puzzle #4

Select the word that is different

G. Dolphin

H. Seal

I. Walrus

J. Cod

K. Turtle

L. Octopus

See page #205 for answers

Brain Exercises

Puzzle #5

Select the word that is different

A. Automobile

B. Truck

C. Bus

D. Monorail

E. Golf Cart

F. Taxi

Puzzle #6

Select the word that is different

G. Ruble

H. Pound

I.   Euro

J. Franc

K. Gold

L. Yen

See page #205 for answers

Brain Exercises Answers

Select the word that is different

PUZZLE	ANSWERS
1. E.	Flower
2. J.	Penguin
3. E.	Porcupine
4. J.	Cod
5. D.	Monorail
6. K.	Gold

Brain Exercises Numbers

Puzzle #7

Select the last number in the series

1   3   6   10   15   21   28   **?**

A. 32

B. 35

C. 30

D. 34

E. 36

Puzzle #8

Select the last number in the series

3   8   6   11   9   14   12   17   15   **?**

F.   22

G.   23

H.   21

I.   18

J.   19

K.   20

Go to page #212 for answers

Brain Exercises Numbers

Puzzle #9

Select the last number in the series

5   13   11   19   17   25   23   **?**

A. 32

B. 31

C. 30

D. 34

E. 21

Puzzle #10

Select the last number in the series

4   8   13   19   26   34   43   53   **?**

F. 62

G. 63

H. 64

I. 65

Go to page #212 for answers

Brain Exercises Numbers

Puzzle #11

Select the last number in the series

11   22   33   44   55   66   77   **?**

A. 86

B. 87

C. 88

D. 89

E. 85

Puzzle #12

Select the last number in the series

5   15   20   30   35   45   50   60   **?**

F.   75

G.   55

H.   70

I.   65

J.   80

Go to page #212 for answers

Brain Exercises Numbers

Puzzle #13

Select the last number in the series

3   6   11   14   19   22   27   30   **?**

A. 38

B. 33

C. 35

D. 37

E. 36

Puzzle #14

Select the last number in the series

550   560   580   590   610   620   640   **?**

F. 655

G. 645

H. 670

I.   660

J.   650

Go to page #212 for answers

Brain Exercises Numbers

Puzzle #15

Select the missing number in the series

70 75 85 90 100 105 115 120 130 **?**

A. 140

B. 135

C. 145

D. 150

E. 155

Puzzle #16

Select the missing number in the series

15 18 21 24 27 30 33 36 39 42 **?**

F. 47

G. 44

H. 49

I. 45

J. 46

Go to page #212 for answers

Brain Exercises Numbers

Puzzle #17

Select the missing number in the series

50 70 100 140 190 250 320 **?**

A. 420

B. 380

C. 390

D. 400

Puzzle #18

Select the missing number in the series

5 9 14 20 27 35 54 64 75 **?**

F. 84

G. 87

H. 82

I. 88

J. 86

Go to page #212 for answers

Brain Exercises Numbers

Determine the last number in the series

Puzzle	Answers
7.	36	Increase each number by previous addition plus one
8.	20	Plus 5, minus 2, repeat
9.	31	Add by eight, minus two, repeat 10.
10.	64	Increase by 4, 5, 6, 7, etc.
11.	88	Plus 11, repeat
12.	65	Plus 10, repeat
13.	35	Plus 3, plus 5, repeat
14.	650	Plus 10, plus 20, repeat
15.	135	Plus 5, plus 10, repeat
16.	45	Plus 3, repeat
17.	400	Plus 10, plus 20, plus 30, plus 40, etc.
18.	87	Plus, add one at each addition

Brain Exercises

Puzzle #19

Unscramble the letters — American Cities

1. L D S A I P N N I O A I

2. I O S N I P N A M E L

3. U S T I G T B R P

4. E O S L E S N L A G

5. N O G T S A W H N I

6. E N A C M O R T A S

Puzzle #20

Unscramble the letters — American Cities

7. B R G A R I H S R U

8. L O R S E C N T A H

9. A S L E T S L A H E A

10. O N G E T O M Y M R

11. E I V N P R E C O D

12. G I A C O C H

Go to page #214 for answers

Brain Exercises
Answers

Puzzle #19

Unscramble the letters — American Cities

1. INDIANAPOLIS

2. MINNEAPOLIS

3. PITTSBURG

4. LOS ANGELES

5. WASHINGTON

6. SACRAMENTO

Puzzle #20

Unscramble the letters — American Cities

G. HARRISBURG

H. CHARLESTON

I. TALLAHASSEE

J. MONTGOMERY

K. PROVIDENCE

L. CHICAGO

Brain Exercises

Puzzle #21

Unscramble the letters — Canadian Cities

1. O L R A E N M T
2. E U R O A V C N
3. A T O W A T
4. T O N M E N D O
5. G I P N I W N E
6. L A X H I A F

Puzzle #22

Unscramble the letters — Canadian Cities

7. N O T T O R O
8. A N F L R L A S G A I A
9. A O K S N O T S A
10. O I R I A V C T
11. E L F O E I Y L W N K
12. O E G B H E P R O T U R

Go to page #216 for answers

Brain Exercises
Answers

Puzzle #21

Unscramble the letters — Canadian Cities

M. MONTREAL

N. VANCOUVER

O. OTTAWA

P. EDMONTON

Q. WINNIPEG

R. HALIFAX

Puzzle #22

Unscramble the letters — Canadian Cities

S. TORONTO

T. NIAGARA FALLS

U. SASKATOON

V. VICTORIA

W. YELLOWKNIFE

X. PETERBOROUGH

Brain Exercises

Puzzle #23

Pair the words, column A with column B
Example: 'High School '

Column A	Column B
Rock	Site
Radio	Game
Real	Coaster
Coffee	Dog
Report	Cream
Hot	Dong
Root	Table
Roller	Account
Web	Glasses
Fish	Skinned
Ice	Ben
Happy	Jack
Dinner	Wave
Thin	Fry
Rocking	Mug
Sun	Minister
Full	Beer
Jumping	Card
Big	Estate
Ding	Belt
Bank	Day
Prime	Horse
Tennis	Band
Life	Court
Video	Moon

Go to page #218 for answers

Brain Exercises
Answers

Puzzle #23

Pair the words, column A with column B
Example: 'High School '

Rock Band
Radio Wave
Real Estate
Coffee Mug
Report Card
Hot Dog
Root Beer
Roller Coaster
Web Site
Fish Fry
Ice Cream
Happy Day
Dinner Table
Thin Skinned
Rocking Horse
Sun Glasses
Full Moon
Jumping Jack
Big Ben
Ding Dong
Bank Account
Prime Minister
Tennis Court
Life Belt
Video Game

Brain Exercises

Puzzle #24

Pair the words, column A with column B
Example: 'Hot Chocolate'

Column A	Column B
Cell	Water
Health	Bag
Oven	Control
Paper	Finger
Dump	Cords
Common	Root
Crossword	President
Bottled	Phone
Rib	Day
Ring	Cleaner
Salad	Mail
Remote	Boots
Sports	Clip
Square	Five
Vacuum	Truck
Valentines	Hearted
Vanilla	Dressing
Vice	Puzzle
High	Room
Waiting	Mitt
Work	Bean
Vocal	Sense
Voice	Drink
Warm	Cage
Sleeping	Care

Go to page #220 for answers

Brain Exercises

Puzzle #24

Pair the words, column A with column B
Example: 'Hot Chocolate '

Cell Phone
Health Care
Oven Mitt
Paper Clip
Dump Truck
Common Sense
Crossword Puzzle
Bottled Water
Rib Cage
Ring Finger
Salad Dressing
Remote Control
Sports Drink
Square Root
Vacuum Cleaner
Valentines day
Vanilla Bean
Vice president
Voice Mail
Vocal Cords
Work Boots
Waiting Room
Sleeping Bag
Warm Hearted
High Five

Brain Exercises

Remember the following names:

Baker, Lawrie, Johnson, Anderson, Peters

Smith, Peterson, Andrews, Rogers, Jackson

Thompson, Handford, Jones, Lewis, Harris

Puzzle #25

Without referencing, select the name which was not included:

A. Jones

B. Thompson

C. Peters

D. Baker

E. Miller

Puzzle #26

Without referencing, select the name which was not included

A. Barnard

B. Rogers

C. Anderson

D. Peterson

E. Johnson

Go to page #227 for answers

Brain Exercises

Remember the following household items:

Basket, pen, microwave, fry pan,

chair, ladder, stool, coffee pot,

telephone, mug, plate, radio

Puzzle #26

Without referencing select the item which was not included:

A. Stool

B. Telephone

C. Flowers

D. Pen

E. Mug

Puzzle #27

Without referencing select the item which was not included:

A. Radio

B. Basket

C. Ladder

D. Can opener

E. Chair

Go to page #227 for answers

Brain Exercises

Remember the following household items:

Basket, pen, microwave, fry pan, bed,

chair, ladder, stool, coffee pot, mop,

telephone, mug, plate, radio, television

Puzzle #28

Without referencing, select the item which was not included:

1. Fry pan

2. Television

3. Mug

4. Coffee Pot

5. Bread box

Puzzle #29

Without referencing, select the item which was not included:

6. Ladder

7. Stapler

8. Chair

9. Rug

10. Mop

Go to page #227 for answers

Brain Exercises

Remember the following household items:

Basket, pen, microwave, fry pan, bed, tea pot

chair, ladder, stool, coffee pot, mop, lawn mower

telephone, mug, plate, radio, television, hammer

Puzzle #30

Without referencing, select the item which was not included:

A. Hammer

B. Television

C. Tea Pot

D. Fan

E. Telephone

Puzzle #31

Without referencing, select the item which was not included:

A. Ladder

B. Heater

C. Chair

D. Rug

E. Fry Pan

Go to page #227 for answers

Brain Exercises

Remember the following names:

Baker, Lawrie, Johnson, Anderson,

Smith, Peterson, Andrews, Rogers

Thompson, Handford, Jones, Lewis

Puzzle #32

Without referencing, select the name which was not included:

1. Rogers
2. Thompson
3. Andrews
4. Foster
5 Lawrie

Puzzle #33

Without referencing, select the name which was not included:

1. Lewis
2. Stewart
3. Handford
4. Peterson
5. Smith

Go to page #227 for answers

Brain Exercises

Remember the following names:

Baker, Lawrie, Johnson, Anderson, Barkwell
Smith, Peterson, Andrews, Rogers, Stacy
Thompson, Handford, Jones, Lewis, Jefferson

Puzzle #34

Without referencing, select the name which was not included:

1. Handford

2. Andrews

3. Adams

4. Stacy

5. Barkwell

Puzzle #35

Without referencing, select the name which was not included:

1. Jones

2. Douglas

3. Jefferson

4. Anderson

5. Smith

Go to page #227 for answers

Brain Exercises
Answers

Puzzle #	Answers
25.	Miller
26.	Barnard
27.	Flowers
28.	Can Opener
29.	Bread Box
30.	Rug
31.	Fan
32.	Heater
33.	Foster
34.	Stewart
35.	Adams
36.	Douglas

Brain Games
Which 3 Numbers Total 200

Puzzle #37

A	B	C	D	E	F	G	H
109	46	82	14	77	68	33	110

Puzzle #38

A	B	C	D	E	F	G	H
78	92	45	121	133	83	67	12

Puzzle #39

A	B	C	D	E	F	G	H
42	86	37	72	104	23	98	24

Puzzle #40

A	B	C	D	E	F	G	H
65	111	39	12	88	45	55	44

Go to page #229 for answers

Brain Games

Answers - Which 3 Total 200

#37 ADE

#38 DGH

#39 DEH

#40 BFH

Retirement Residences (1)

Thoughtfully designed retirement residences are being introduced across the United States, Canada, Australia and most European countries. These facilities offer security, comfort and encourage a lifestyle of social and brain stimulating activities. The following features commonly found in retirement   residences:

Brain Wellness Programs

Fitness Center / Spa
Brain Stimulating Programs
Library / Book Clubs
Social Games / Puzzle Challenges
Poem and Limerick Groups
Memory Programs
DVD / Netflix Movies
Music Participation
DVD Concerts
Dancing / Live Music Entertainment

Services

Shuttle Bus for Outings
Convenience Shop
Beauty Hair Styling Shop

Weekly Housekeeping Service
Weekly Linen and Towel Service

Retirement Residences (2)

Safety and Security

24 Hour Security

Reception Entry

Emergency Response Pendants

Intercom Systems in Each Suite

Sprinkler Systems and Smoke Detectors

Wheelchair Accessible

Bathroom Safety Features

Safe Parking Areas

Special Features

24 Hour Management and Wellness Staff

On-Site Nurse and Caregivers

Warm Comfortable Atmosphere

Kitchenettes

Spacious Apartments and Bathrooms

Individual Climate Controls

Connections for Phone and Cablevision

Beauty Shop / Barber Shop

Private Mail Boxes

Park like Landscaping

Hospitality Suites

On-Site Chapel

Elegant Dining Room

Delicious Balance Meals

Coffee Shops Featuring Pastries

Friday Night Happy Hour

Dementia Villages

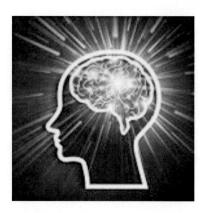

Parkway Villages (1)
Creative Dementia Housing

A creative new form of housing for those dealing with dementia disorders is now being introduced in several countries. The objective, to create a warm comfortable atmosphere similar to what would be found back home in a typical city or town. The objective is to build an atmosphere where there is the potential to slow or reverse dementia disorders.

These new residences have been designed and built based on a large common indoor area where you will find walkways similar to a park bordered by imitation trees and grass. Along the path there are lanterns, live flowers, plants and bushes. Park benches under the lanterns provide a friendly warm comforting atmosphere. Individual apartments as you enter resemble small cottages with inviting porches.

In the large common area a variety of familiar games are offered including a putting green, shuffle board and miniature bocce ball, lawn bowling along with other fun popular games and activities. Tables with chairs invite card and board games. A comfortable seating area where soothing music is piped in inviting the residents to relax, avoid stress and simply enjoy the day in this warm wonderful setting.

Parkway Villages (2)

In the common room, windows border along the top of the exterior high wall allowing natural light to shine into the area during the day. At night the blue ceiling provides sparkling stars a beautiful colorful moon together with soothing music.

The hallways are built to resemble streets which lead to the cottage like homes and a row of shops all with actual store fronts. They include a candy store a coffee/pastry shop, a theatre, a church, a library, a barber shop/hair stylist, a general products shop, all designed to resemble main street in a small village. The street also includes the nurse and wellness directors offices.

A cooking club has been organized to encourage those who miss their home baking. Several people can join together to bake tasty treats. They mix and bake, have fun and enjoy great conversation.

Parkway Villages (3)

The common area also includes a stage and a dance floor. Musicians are provided, often sponsored by local businesses. Residents are encouraged to dance or sing along to old favorites. In Holland a pianist may play old songs that are familiar such as 'Edel-weiss', 'O Sle Mio', 'Moon River' or other favorites. It is very common for the audience to sing along.

If they can, residents begin to dance, they stand up from their chairs, holding hands with aides and shifting slowly from side to side. An elderly woman with a gray braid and joyful expression walked to the middle of the floor but then stopped to listen to the piano, and began to sway to the music.

The theatre provides entertaining movies three times a week. Daily brain stimulating workshops provide challenging memory programs. The staff encourage residents to attend and take part. These workshops are proving to reverse or stabilize dementia in most cases.

At one location, a one acre outdoor park has been built with fully fenced facilities. These include gardens, a cookery or pizza oven where the resident can make snacks and serve treats while they all enjoy the outdoors.

Parkway Villages (4)

In all locations the family dog or cat is in residence and they provide love and comfort for those needing the attention, that only a beloved pet can provide.

Each apartment is just like a home which includes a shingled roof, a large window, a front door with a street address and a mail box. Most homes feature a small porch to enhance the home. Rocking chairs encourage the resident and family visitors to sit and chat. In the evening as it begins to grow dark outside, lights on the porches and the pathway lanterns give a feeling of warmth.

The Village concept encourages residents to become involved in this unique community. The Villages are proving to discourage isolation which is a common problem even in the finest retirement residences where typically 20% to 40% of the population seldom leave their apartments. Lack of social connection advances dementia.

The village concept provides a new and advanced opportunity to reverse or delay dementia.

60 Reinforcements

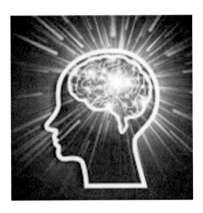

60 Reinforcements

1. Test your recall — make a list of grocery items or things to do, or anything else that can force recall. Make items on the list as challenging as possible for the greatest mental stimulation. Now, on a separate piece of paper write the list backwards.

2. Learn to play a musical instrument and make it challenging but also enjoyable. A home style electric organ can be real fun, a small piano, a guitar or a harmonica.

3. Learn something new and more complex over a longer period of time.

4. Do math in your head. Figure out problems without a calculator, or a pencil, make it more challenging by walking briskly while solving the calculation.

5. Take a cooking class. Learn how to cook something exotic or a delicious soup. Make it a special treat.

6. Learn a new language. Listening and hearing involved in language training will stimulate the brain.

60 Reinforcements

7. Create word pictures. Visualize the spelling of a word in your head, try to think of other words with a similar meaning.

8. Draw maps from memory.

9. Challenge your taste buds when eating. Identify individual ingredients. Have friends over for a taste testing contest.

10. Take up knitting. Test your mind and hand motor skills.

11. Learn a new sport, golf, tennis, lawn bowling, or pickle ball.

12. Be a constant reader, set a goal to read a book a week. Buy a Kindle or an alternate reading tablet.

13. Always be an attentive listener.

14. Start or join an on-line joke club (print, images and videos).

15. Join a choir.

16. Smile when talking on the telephone.

17.Write down three positive things each day.

60 Reinforcements

18. Memorize the words to songs. Most lyrics are available online and can be printed. Consider buying the matching CD or DVD and then sing along.

19. Take a neighbor's dog for a walk.

20. Become an author, write a story or a fun complimentary 'Limerick' about your good friend. Print the limerick and send by post mail with a friendship card.

21. Play brain games online. Search your local library for books with brain games or brain facts.

22. Write a book about your life, connect with a 'Life's Journey Group.'

23. Read books or the newspaper OUT LOUD.

24. Play scrabble with family, join a community card club.

25. Rent a plot, grow a vegetable garden which includes some brain vegetables.

26. Challenge yourself to a new adventure.

27. Take some flowers to an older person or someone ill.

28. Let go of negative thoughts.

60 Reinforcements

29. Take up painting, attend a class.

30. Join a bicycle club and tour your town or city.

31. Join a Miniature Club. Create miniature homes.

32. Become a story teller, read to seniors or children.

33. Play billiards, develop better hand and eye coordination. .

34. Extend your memory. Start with something not too extensive.

35. Name all the bones in your body.

36. Name the characters in your favorite movie or TV show.

37. Regularly put a little money in a separate savings account.

38. Name the characters in your favorite funny movie.

39. Take dancing lessons.

40. Go for a walk as often as possible and count your steps.

41. List and remember the birth dates of the ten people you enjoy the most. Send a birthday card.

42. Every week give someone a gift. Find a lonely person and make their day. A gift for a co-worker, the newspaper delivery person, your doctor's receptionist this will make you feel good.

60 Reinforcements

43. Be kind to strangers.

44. Stop accepting plastic bags, cups or straws.

45. Praise, encourage and congratulate

46. Stop eating harmful foods.

47. Never speed when driving.

48. Always be patient, never honk your horn.

49. Slow down and let someone in your lane when driving.

50. Write down a list of your ten neighbors.

51. Keep a daily record of who, what, where and why.

52. Be confident and love yourself.

53. Control your blood pressure.

54. Watch your weight.

55. Drink alcohol in moderation.

56. Give a sincere compliment.

57. Love your brain. It is the only one you will ever have.

58. Bring positivity to a discussion.

59. Say 'Thank You' like you really mean it.

60. Leave a note on the mirror, tell him or her you love them.

Acknowledgements

We hope this book will encourage everyone to use this book as a wellness guide to prevent, delay or reverse the onset of dementia brain disorders. I urge everyone to make a commitment to expand your social life and exercise their brain each and every day.

My sincere appreciation to my wife Yvonne, my two daughters Alexandria and Ava, my amazing two good friends Ron Stenning and Morris Dorosh all who have provided support and guidance in creating this publication.

I thank Cheryl, Chantal, Jillian, Donovan, Jackie, and Brandi who have hosted Mind & Memory workshops presented at their retirement residences. My thanks to Linda Fischer and Marilyn McKellar for detailed editing. To all the ladies at Seine River Retirement Residence, Jeannie Kostick, Irene Hodgson, Wilma Harrison, Irene Peters, Doreen Tough, Irene Nuytten, and Edna Butler who leant support and made valued suggestions. Thanks to the Military Legions, Seniors Clubs, Credit Unions and Medical centers who hosted our workshops. Whose members and guests recognize the importance of fighting this mind altering brain disorder.

Gary Adams

Author and Publisher

About the author

Gary G. Adams

After a successful 30 years developing condominium communities, suddenly Gary recognized that his key sales associate and close friend had dementia disorder, was loosing his memory and becoming disoriented. Gary then turned his attention to creating workshops to stimulate mind and memory.

For over a decade Gary has provided brain stimulating exercises for seniors' as well as those in mid-life. His Mind and Memory Workshops have helped hundreds of people retain and nourish their brains and potentially avoid dementia.

While presenting his brain enhancing programs, Gary has experienced first hand how those who are socially and physically active have avoided dementia. He also observed that dementia disorder is primarily caused by social and brain inactivity (a lazy brain) and strongly believes dementia can, with determination, be prevented or stabilized.

People are living much longer. As they age a high percentage of people become isolated. A disinterested attitude and a lazy brain are key factors in the rapid increase of dementia.

Gary encourages everyone, as they age to practice daily brain defense exercises starting in mid-life.